Zana Kadir

# The effectiveness of physiotherapy in the treatment of patients with CMD

Zana Kadir

# The effectiveness of physiotherapy in the treatment of patients with CMD

## A systematic review based on randomized controlled trials

ScienciaScripts

**Imprint**
Any brand names and product names mentioned in this book are subject to trademark, brand or patent protection and are trademarks or registered trademarks of their respective holders. The use of brand names, product names, common names, trade names, product descriptions etc. even without a particular marking in this work is in no way to be construed to mean that such names may be regarded as unrestricted in respect of trademark and brand protection legislation and could thus be used by anyone.

Cover image: www.ingimage.com

This book is a translation from the original published under ISBN 978-620-8-86943-4.

Publisher:
Sciencia Scripts
is a trademark of
Dodo Books Indian Ocean Ltd. and OmniScriptum S.R.L publishing group

120 High Road, East Finchley, London, N2 9ED, United Kingdom
Str. Armeneasca 28/1, office 1, Chisinau MD-2012, Republic of Moldova, Europe
Managing Directors: Ieva Konstantinova, Victoria Ursu
info@omniscriptum.com

Printed at: see last page
**ISBN: 978-620-8-99227-9**

Contents

# FOREWORD

The path seems rocky - you feel insecure and overwhelmed at first, but an inner voice calls out: "You can do it, keep going." You find the connection, join the ranks of your fellow travellers and continue on your way. The journey may seem long, but at some point you reach your goal - only to realise that it might not be the final destination after all.

This is the path I have chosen - a journey into the uncharted territory of science. It is the desire to achieve something greater.

I don't know how far I want to or can go. But curiosity drives me on and the thought of what's to come won't let me go. It's probably the secret of scientific work: once you start, you simply can't stop.

## ACKNOWLEDGEMENTS / DEDICATIONS

My heartfelt thanks go to all those who have always believed in me and supported me. I would also like to say a big thank you to my university, its staff and the lecturers from whom I was able to gain valuable insights.

I would especially like to thank my supervisor, Mr Rainer Schwarz, who provided me with advice and support during my Master's thesis. I would also like to emphasise Mrs Dangl and Mrs Tüchler, who motivated me to keep going in the initial phase when I was on the verge of giving up. Finally, I would like to thank David Schardt and Philipp Riebe for their support in the moments when I needed it most.

## BRIEF DESCRIPTION

**Problem:** Tinnitus is a considerable burden for those affected, as it is not only annoying and prolonged, but is often accompanied by hearing loss. For doctors and therapists, treatment proves to be challenging, especially when tinnitus is associated with craniomandibular dysfunction (CMD) or disorders of the upper cervical spine (cervical spine) - a phenomenon that is referred to in the specialist literature as somatosensory tinnitus. The treatment of somatosensory tinnitus requires a sound diagnosis and interdisciplinary collaboration between different medical specialities. These disciplines include physiotherapy, dentistry, ear, nose and throat medicine, psychotherapy, pharmacology, orthopaedics and orthodontics. Studies suggest that physiotherapy can be an effective treatment option in these cases.

**Study design**: This systematic review is based on the analysis of ten randomised controlled trials (RCTs) investigating the effectiveness of physiotherapeutic interventions for somatosensory tinnitus.

**Results:** The studies analysed show that physiotherapy has a significant effect on patients with somatosensory tinnitus both as a stand-alone treatment and as part of multimodal approaches. The results include a reduction in tinnitus distress (e.g. measured by the Tinnitus Handicap Inventory [THI] and visual analogue scales [VAS]) as well as improvements in functional and emotional parameters.

**Conclusion**: In this master's thesis, the effectiveness of physiotherapy for tinnitus associated with CMD or upper cervical spine disorders is demonstrated by analysing the selected ten RCTs. The literature emphasises the central role of physiotherapy, particularly as part of a multidisciplinary approach, in alleviating tinnitus symptoms and improving quality of life. However, methodological weaknesses in the study situation, such as the small number of high-quality RCTs, small samples and short follow-up periods, emphasise the need for further high-quality, large-scale RCTs in order to further strengthen the evidence base and to investigate and prove the long-term effectiveness of specific physiotherapy approaches, both in comparison and as an add-on therapy to other interventions.



**Keywords (author keywords):** Physiotherapy, interventions, temporomandibular joint, craniomandibular dysfunction (CMD), temporomandibular dysfunction (TMD), tinnitus, somatosensory tinnitus, cervical spine (cervical spine), upper cervical spine and randomised controlled trials (RCTs).

CHAPTER 1

# 1 Introduction

## Background

Miyamoto et al. (2024, cited in Stulin et al., 2021, and Henry et al., 2020) explain that the term "tinnitus" is derived from the Latin word "tinnire", which means "to ring like a bell". They describe tinnitus as an otological manifestation (cited in Palmer & Durham, 2021) caused by a reaction of the central nervous system (cited in Stulin et al., 2021), the limbic system and the autonomic nervous system (cited in Henry et al., 2020). This disorder manifests itself through the perception of buzzing or ringing sounds that can vary in intensity (cited in Australian et al., 2015).

Koporal et al (2022) define tinnitus as the perception of sounds that are not triggered by external acoustic stimuli and point out that it affects around 10-15% of the population. According to them, there are many factors that can trigger tinnitus, such as trauma, otological and neurological problems, side effects of medication, inflammatory diseases, depression and temporomandibular joint disorders (cited in Gelb et al., 1997). They emphasise that tinnitus is often caused by interactions in the somatosensory system of the central nervous system. Sometimes, however, tinnitus is also caused directly by disturbances in the head and neck area when this system is activated. In addition, somatic factors outside the ear, such as temporomandibular joint disorders, can contribute to the development of tinnitus (Koporal et al., 2022).

According to Henry et al (2013), the severity of tinnitus can be expressed by the health-related quality of life (measured with the Tinnitus Functional Index, TFI) and the loudness of the tinnitus (assessed with the visual analogue scale, VAS), as there are no objective methods for measuring tinnitus.

According to Meulemeester et al. (2023, cited in De Ridder et al., 2021), subjective tinnitus is the most common form and occurs in 95% of all patients. It is defined as "the conscious perception of a tonal or compound sound for which there is no recognisable external acoustic source." When subjective tinnitus is triggered by the somatosensory system of the cervical spine or temporomandibular joint, it is referred to as somatic tinnitus (Michiels et al., 2018; cf. Baguley et al., 2013; Axelsson & Ringdahl, 1989).

Sanchez and Rocha (2011 b,c) describe that signs of somatosensory tinnitus include problems in the head or neck area, such as temporomandibular joint syndrome, osteoarthritis, spondylosis, osteophytes and myofascial trigger points. Dental or jaw diseases, frequent pain in the head, neck or shoulder area, unphysiological postures, severe bruxism and an aggravation of symptoms with concurrent pain and tinnitus are also mentioned as relevant indicators.

Michiels et al. (2018) emphasise that the complexity of these relationships often requires a team of specialists, such as dentists and physiotherapists, to work together. Langguth et al. (2024), citing Michiels et al. (2018), Kreuzer et al. (2014) and Shore et al. (2016), explain that there are several indications of the involvement of the somatosensory system in tinnitus.

Michiels et al (2018) state that "the majority of tinnitus patients can modulate their tinnitus by moving their head". Kreuzer et al. (2014) add that tinnitus is more common in patients with temporomandibular joint disorders and in some cases is triggered by neck trauma, such as whiplash.

In their systematic review, Bousema et al. (2018) described various models to explain subjective somatosensory tinnitus in connection with temporomandibular joint disorders. One frequently mentioned model assumes that "a disorder of the temporomandibular joint, such as a disc displacement, or hypertonia of the masticatory muscles through anatomical connections, such as the tensor veli palatini, the Eustachian tube or several ligaments, can influence the tension or ventilation of the middle ear muscles". "These influences would generate afferent signals that - via the cochlear nerve - would influence the auditory pathways" (Ramirez et al., 2008).

According to Shore and Zhou (2006), recent studies have identified a connection between the trigeminal and dorsal column systems of the somatosensory system and the cochlear nucleus (CN) of the auditory system in the medulla oblongata. Shore (2011) explains that the spinal trigeminal nucleus "receives nociceptive and proprioceptive input from the head, face, oral structures, temporomandibular joint and cervical spine (C1-C3) and projects to the cochlear nucleus". According to Shore (2005), one function of this connection may be to distinguish between external sounds and those produced by the body.

According to Da Silva et al. (2023, cited in Vielsmeier et al., 2012), an increase in temporomandibular joint symptoms from 19% to 36% was found in a group of test subjects with severe tinnitus. This suggests that temporomandibular joint pain, muscle tension, teeth grinding, jaw clenching and chewing difficulties can contribute to the worsening of tinnitus (Da Silva et al., 2023, cited in Vielsmeier et al., 2012; Edvall et al., 2019). Treatment that targets these complaints could therefore be helpful for patients with tinnitus and temporomandibular joint disorders, as this could be considered a separate subtype of tinnitus (Da Silva et al., 2023, cited in Edvall et al., 2019).

According to Lomas et al. (2018, cited after Sharma et al., 2011), CMD comprises a group of disorders of the masticatory system that are roughly divided into muscular disorders and disorders of the temporomandibular joint (TMJ). CMD is a widespread disorder that affects up to 60-70% of the population. The highest incidence occurs in adults aged between 20 and 40 years, with women being affected about four times more frequently than men. Despite the high prevalence of CMD, symptomatic forms requiring treatment only occur in around 5% to 12% of the population (Lomas et al., 2018, cited in National Institute of Dental and Craniofacial Research, 2014). In general, according to Lomas et al., CMD refers to pain in the temporomandibular joint and surrounding structures as well as dysfunction of the joint itself.

Gçbska et al. (2023, cited in Casañas et al. 2021; Raya et al. 2017) describe in their study that CMDs are not only related to the temporomandibular joints (TMJ) and the masticatory muscles, but are also often associated with other health problems in the head and neck area, such as headaches, ear symptoms and cervical spine dysfunction. According to Michiels et al. (2014), cervicogenic somatic tinnitus is a subtype that is triggered by cervical spine dysfunction and therefore warrants assessment and treatment of the cervical spine.

According to Biesinger et al. (2015), Decher pointed out in his monograph as early as 1962 that tinnitus could be caused or triggered by structural and functional pathologies of the cervical spine. At that time, according to Biesinger et al., these findings were primarily based on clinical observations and individual case descriptions.

In their RCT, Michiels et al. (2016) pointed out the high number of patients with CST, which was reported in earlier studies (Abel & Levine, 2004; Fabijanska et al., 2014; Ostermann et al., 2014; Michiels et al., 2015) as 36-43 % of all tinnitus patients. Patients with CST often suffer from limited rotation of the cervical spine (Reisshauer et al., 2006; Michiels et al., 2015), pain provocation with simultaneous extension, lateral tilt and rotation of the cervical spine (Michiels et al, 2015) or sensitive trigger points (Reisshauer et al., 2006; Michiels et al., 2015), especially if they achieve a score of more than 14/70 on the Neck Bournemouth Questionnaire (NBQ) (Michiels et al., 2015).

Wadhwa et al. (2024, cited in Sajadi et al., 2019) describe that the pathophysiology of CST is complex and is based on the interplay between somatosensory impulses from the cervical spine and the central auditory pathways. This pathophysiology is characterised by strong contractions of the jaw and neck muscles, which influence the psychoacoustic properties of

the tinnitus.
Kaltenbach (2005) considers CST to be a special form of somatic tinnitus. The involvement of the spinal ganglia of the second, seventh and eighth cervical nerves and the trigeminal ganglion is considered crucial for the connections to the auditory system. Changes in brainstem structures associated with hearing and influenced by cervical inputs may contribute to the development of CST.
According to Bousema et al. (2023), physiotherapy is playing an increasingly important role in the treatment of subjective tinnitus. Physical therapies used include transcutaneous electrical nerve stimulation (TENS), laser therapy, the treatment of temporomandibular joint disorders, acupuncture, biofeedback and kinesio-taping, according to Bousema et al. However, the scientific basis for some of these methods, such as acupuncture, is not always clear. According to Shore and Zhou (2006), therapies such as TENS, laser therapy or the treatment of temporomandibular joint dysfunction are based on the assumption that somatosensory stimuli can influence the auditory system through connections between the cochlear nucleus and the trigeminal and spinal systems.
This connection could explain why many sufferers can influence their tinnitus loudness and pitch by tensing their neck, head or jaw muscles (Bjorne, 2007; Bonaconsa et al, 2010; Levine, 1999; Pinchoff et al, 1998; Rocha & Sanchez, 2007; Rubinstein, 1993; Sanchez et al, 2002; Vernon et al, 1992). It has also been shown that tinnitus patients suffer more frequently from disorders of the cervical spine or temporomandibular joint. Studies report a 2.6 to 6.7-fold increased risk in these groups (Omidvar & Jafari, 2019; Mottaghi et al., 2019; Bousema et al., 2018).
According to Urbariski et al. (2021, cited in Okeson, 2013), the effectiveness of CMD treatment depends on eliminating the causes responsible for the dysfunction of the temporomandibular system. According to Urbariski et al., direct intervention in the muscles is important to restore their natural tension and relieve pain. Clinicians and researchers recommend using conservative treatments first before considering irreversible methods (Okeson, 2013; D'Attilio et al., 2021; Liu & Steinkeler, 2013).
Current approaches in CMD treatment include prosthetic and orthodontic measures (Okeson, 2013; D'Attilio et al., 2021; Liu & Steinkeler, 2013) as well as the use of medication (Okeson, 2013; Pihut et al., 2016; Mor et al., 2015). One of the most commonly recommended conservative therapies is physiotherapy, including manual techniques (Asquini et al, 2019; De Resende et al, 2019; Brochado et al, 2018; Pessoa et al, 2018; Pablo Delgado et al, 2019;
Reynolds et al, 2020; Tuncer et al, 2013; Wieckiewicz et al, 2015). The combined use of these procedures with prosthetic treatment can significantly accelerate the restoration of normal function of the masticatory apparatus (Okeson, 2013; DeToledo et al., 2012; Biegariska, 2016).
Chaitow (2015) and Ballantyne et al. (2003) explain that post-isometric relaxation (PIR) is a favoured technique in manual therapy. It is based on neurophysiological mechanisms and ensures that muscles relax immediately after an isometric contraction. This can reduce muscle-related pain.
The MR technique works by relaxing the myofascial system and helps to relieve tension and pain (Chaitow & Delany, 2008; Manheim et al, 2011; Myers et al, 2012; Cantu & Grodin, 2001).

## Relevance and objectives

Based on the summarised findings from the literature on tinnitus, CMD and functional disorders of the upper cervical spine, it can be said that these disorders are associated with considerable suffering and a significant reduction in quality of life for those affected. They also represent a major challenge for physiotherapists and other medical professionals because they often require lengthy and complex therapeutic approaches due to the combination of physical, psychological and social stress. A purely symptom-orientated treatment is usually not enough.

It becomes particularly problematic when tinnitus persists over a longer period of time, as this causes hearing loss and increases the risk of it becoming chronic. CMD is similarly complex, as its effects often extend beyond the cranial regions of the body and can cause secondary disorders in other areas. Patients who suffer from tinnitus, CMD or dysfunctions of the upper cervical spine at the same time are often faced with a particularly stressful situation from which they can hardly escape on their own and are dependent on various therapeutic approaches, which almost always include physiotherapy as a supplementary component.

The aim of this paper is to investigate, based on a literature review, how patients with somatosensory tinnitus can best be helped and what contribution physiotherapy can make as an independent or complementary therapy.

CHAPTER 2

# 2 Theoretical framework

In accordance with the topics formulated in the research question, this work comprises the following main components: Physiotherapy, CMD, temporomandibular joint, cervical spine and tinnitus.

## 2.1 Physiotherapy

According to Michiels et al. (2017), physiotherapy is a simple, non-invasive and easily accessible treatment option. Bousema et al. (2023) report that more and more people with subjective tinnitus are visiting physiotherapists to receive therapies such as transcutaneous electrical nerve stimulation (TENS), laser therapy, acupuncture, orofacial therapy, kinesio-taping and biofeedback.

In the treatment of CMD, physiotherapy aims to alleviate the symptoms and restore the normal function of the masticatory system (Pelicioli et al., 2017). Techniques such as laser, ultrasound or cathodic current are used. Manual therapy also plays an important role and includes muscle stretching exercises, joint mobilisation and exercises to stabilise the cervical spine (Amaral et al., 2013; Freitas et al., 2011; Calixtre et al., 2016; Franco et al., 2011).

Gil-Martinez et al. (2018, cited in McNeely et al., 2006; Medlicott & Harris, 2006; Sturdivant & Fricton, 1991) emphasise that physiotherapy plays an important role in the treatment of CMD. The aim is to relieve pain, reduce inflammation and improve mobility through various techniques. These include manual therapy such as joint mobilisation and soft tissue techniques, therapeutic exercises and electrotherapy. Examples of electrotherapy include low-level laser therapy (LLLT), transcutaneous electrical nerve stimulation (TENS), ultrasound treatments and short waves. Dry needling and acupuncture are also often used (McNeely et al., 2006; Paço et al., 2016).

Gçbska et al. (2023, cited in Rocabado et al., 2021; von Piekartz et al., 2021) emphasise the importance of cooperation between dentists and physiotherapists in the diagnosis of CMDs. This cooperation makes it possible to make early diagnoses and significantly improve the effectiveness of therapeutic measures. Advances in science and wider access to specialised services have led to physiotherapy for CMDs becoming increasingly important. Numerous studies, including those by Rocabado and Piekartz, have established dental physiotherapy as a dynamic and promising speciality.

Latifpour et al (2009) conducted an RCT with 13 tinnitus patients and 11 control subjects. They found a significant improvement in tinnitus loudness after the application of stretching exercises, postural exercises and acupuncture compared to the control group ($p < 0.001$). The intervention comprised physiotherapy treatment of the cervical spine, including manual mobilisation, movement therapy and home exercises. This multimodal physiotherapy is based on current evidence for the treatment of the cervical spine (cited in Gross et al., 2004; Kay et al., 2012; Miller et al., 2010).

According to Michiels et al. (2014, cited in Miller et al., 2011; Kay et al., 2012; Cleland et al., 2010), recent studies show that multimodal physiotherapy programmes that combine mobilisation or manipulation with exercise therapy achieve better results than treatments that are limited to mobilisation or manipulation alone.

## 2.2 Craniomandibular dysfunction (CMD)

### 2.2.1 Definition of terms

According to Ahmad et al (2021), CMDs encompass a variety of disorders affecting the temporomandibular joint (TMJ), the masticatory muscles and the associated structural system. The most common forms include myofascial pain, internal joint dysfunction and degenerative joint disease. CMDs usually have a multifactorial aetiology and treatment options range from conservative therapies to surgical interventions.

### 2.2.2 Aetiology

According to Lomas et al. (2018, cited after Sharma et al., 2011), the aetiology of CMD is multifactorial and includes anatomical, pathophysiological and psychosocial factors. According to the authors, successful treatment requires the identification and treatment of these predisposing and contributing factors. According to La Hernández-Nuño et al. (2022, cited in Levine, 1999), the understanding of CMD aetiology has evolved from a purely anatomical approach to a biopsychosocial model that takes into account the complexity of these chronic pain disorders. Studies on the frequency of otological symptoms in patients with CMD show that a feeling of ear pressure (74.8%) is the most common symptom, followed by ear pain (55.1%), tinnitus (52.1%), dizziness (40.8%) and hearing loss (La Hernández-Nuño et al., 2022, cited in Baguley et al., 2013).

Lomas et al. (cited in Reiter et al., 2012) point out that it is important to differentiate between myofascial causes of CMD and problems in the temporomandibular joint itself. Myofascial disorders are caused by muscle tension, overload or spasms, while problems in the joint are more likely to be due to mechanical or inflammatory causes. According to Lomas et al. (cited in Reiter et al., 2012), musculoskeletal problems are the most common cause of CMD.

Behaviours such as teeth grinding, teeth clenching or poor posture, as well as stress and anxiety, can trigger muscle pain and spasms in the jaw. In addition, psychological problems such as depression and anxiety disorders as well as autoimmune diseases, fibromyalgia and other chronic pain are often associated with CMD, according to Lomas et al. (cited in Scrivani et al., 2008). This could indicate that the complaints are part of a larger pain syndrome.

Lomas et al. (cited in de Leeuw & Klasser, 2013) describe the intra-articular causes of CMD. These include internal joint disorders, osteoarthritis, inflammation of the joint capsule, excessive mobility (hypermobility) and injuries caused by accidents. Inflammatory diseases such as rheumatoid arthritis or ankylosing spondylitis can also cause such problems. Displacement of the joint disc from its normal position is the most common intra-articular cause of CMD. Lomas et al. also emphasise that disc displacement often causes no symptoms in many people. In addition, there is little evidence that misalignment of the teeth (occlusal disorders) can trigger CMD.

### 2.2.3 Clinical patterns

Gil-Martinez (2018, cited in Suvinen et al., 2005) describes pain as one of the most common symptoms of CMD. This pain often affects the ears, eyes or throat and can also cause neck, facial and head pain. Physical causes include inflammatory problems such as traumatic secondary synovitis, infection and irritation (Graff-Radford, 2007).

According to Da Silva et al. (2023, cited in Conti et al., 2012; Costa et al., 2016; Silveira et al., 2015; Porto et al., 2017), localised or diffuse orofacial pain is the main symptom of CMD. Other common symptoms include joint noises, restricted mouth opening, neck pain, headaches and otological complaints such as tinnitus, hyperacusis, dizziness and balance disorders.

According to Delgado et al. (2020, cited in Algieri et al., 2017), tinnitus is a common symptom of CMD. Both CMD and tinnitus typically occur in the fifth decade of life and affect women more frequently than men at a ratio of 3:2. Studies show that patients with CMD suffer from tinnitus more frequently than those without CMD (Delgado et al., 2020, cited in Kim et al., 2018). Conversely, people with tinnitus are also more likely to develop symptoms associated with CMD ( Delgado et al., 2020, cited in Song et al., 2018).

### 2.2.4 Diagnostics

According to Li and Leung (2021), the most important step in the diagnosis of CMD is to distinguish common conditions from less common but clinically significant conditions and from more serious conditions that require immediate treatment. Some tumours, such as chondrosarcoma of the temporomandibular joint, may initially present with symptoms such as

pain in the preauricular area or restricted mouth opening, which are similar to typical CMD diagnoses. Another example is temporal arteritis, which is a
Inflammation of the temporal arteries, which can cause symptoms similar to CMD, such as headaches, pain in the temple area and restricted mouth opening. However, this condition is a medical emergency as it can lead to permanent blindness if left untreated.

2.2.5 Differential diagnoses (DD)

Li and Leung (2021) provide a comprehensive overview of the DD of CMD, which includes the following categories:

- □ Neuropathic pain: Trigeminal neuralgia, Traumatic neuralgia Glossopharyngeal neuralgia, Postherpetic neuralgia, Burning mouth syndrome, Atypical odontalgia, Atypical facial pain
- □ Odontogenic pain: dental caries, periodontal disease, dental abscess, dental sensitivity, cracked tooth syndrome, pericoronitis
- □ Intracranial pain: tumours, aneurysms, bleeding, infections
- □ Pain from neighbouring structures: ears, nose, throat, eyes, sinuses, salivary glands, lymph nodes, vascular system, cervical spine
- □ Headaches that are not caused by CMD: Migraine, cluster headaches, tension headaches, temporal arteritis
- □ Transmitted pain
- □ Psychogenic pain

These categories reflect a modified version of the work by Kumar et al. (2013).

2.2.6 Therapeutic approaches

According to Da Silva et al. (2023, cited in Vielsmeier et al., 2012; Mottaghi et al., 2019; Vielsmeier et al., 2011; Gauer & Semidey, 2015; Gil-Martinez et al., 2018), a multidisciplinary approach is crucial for the treatment of CMD. These disorders can impair quality of life and lead to sleep disorders, anxiety, stress and mood swings. There is evidence that conservative treatments, particularly PT, can help to improve symptoms and mandibular mobility in patients with CMD (Da Silva et al., 2023, cited in Gil-Martinez et al., 2018; McNeely et al., 2006).

According to Gil-Martinez et al. (2018, cited in Gauer & Semidey, 2015), an appropriate therapeutic approach to CMD should aim to alleviate the main signs and symptoms of the condition. The most common symptoms include joint sounds such as clicking or crepitation, restricted mouth opening and disturbed jaw movements (Suvinen et al., 2005; Dworkin et al., 1990). However, pain is the main problem with CMD, which usually leads patients to seek medical help (Gil-Martinez et al., 2018, cited in Ghurye & McMillan, 2015; Oral et al., 2009). As a result, many studies have attempted to investigate the effectiveness of different treatment methods in terms of pain reduction (Gil-Martinez et al., 2018, cited in Fricton et al., 2010).

In their study published in 2018, Gil-Martinez et al. report on various treatment approaches for CMD patients, based on the work of Ingawalé & Goswami (2009), McNeely et al. (2006), Medlicott & Harris (2006), Paço et al. (2016), Scrivani et al. (2008) and Liste & Axelsson (2010). They point out that conservative treatments are currently favoured over surgical interventions as they are non-invasive and generally provide good clinical results in mild to moderate CMD (Scrivani et al., 2008; Syrop, 2002; Dimitroulis et al., 1995; Armijo et al., 2016). These include the following treatment approaches:

- □ Conservative treatment: This includes medication, PT, occlusal splints, self-management strategies and interventions based on cognitive behavioural therapies.
- □ Oral and topical pharmacotherapy: non-steroidal anti-inflammatory drugs (NSAIDs), corticosteroids, analgesics, muscle relaxants, anxiolytics, opiates, tricyclic antidepressants

(TCAs), gabapentin and lidocaine patches are most commonly used (Agjus et al, 2013; Weißer et al, 2011; Gewandter et al, 2011; Firmani et al, 2015).

□ Injected pharmacotherapy: A recent review shows that injections of corticosteroid ß-methasone or sodium hyaluronate are effective in the treatment of TMJ pain (Liste & Axelsson, 2010; Häggman et al., 2017).

□ Surgical interventions

□ Dental management: Dentists usually offer two therapeutic approaches: orthopaedic stabilisation therapy and occlusal therapy to improve jaw function (Armijo et al., 2016).

□ Physiotherapy: This plays a central role in CMD treatment and aims to reduce pain, relieve inflammation and restore motor function. The techniques used include manual therapy (e.g. joint mobilisation and soft tissue mobilisation), therapeutic exercises, electrotherapy (e.g. low-level laser therapy [LLLT], transcutaneous electrical nerve stimulation [TENS], ultrasound), dry needling and acupuncture (McNeely et al., 2006; Medlicott & Harris, 2006).

□ Manual therapy: This includes techniques for mobilising joints and soft tissues to improve function and relieve pain (Calixtre et al., 2015; Armijo et al., 2016).

□ Therapeutic exercises: Exercises to improve motor control and endurance of the masticatory muscles have been shown to be effective in relieving CMD symptoms (Armijo et al., 2016).

□ Dry needling (ND) and acupuncture: Only a few studies were found that used DN for CMD (Fernández-Carnero et al, 2010; González-Iglesias et al, 2013; Gonzalez-Perez et al, 2015; Blasco-Bonora & Martín-Pintado-Zugasti, 2017). This intervention is used to treat localised and referred pain caused by myofascial trigger points (Simons & Travell, 1999).

□ Electrotherapy (ET): The evidence for the use of ET for pain relief in CMD is limited (McNeely et al., 2006; Liste & Axelsson, 2010).

□ Cognitive behavioural therapy

□ Educational and self-management strategies: These strategies, when combined with other techniques, such as MT, can effectively alleviate CMD symptoms (Michelotti et al., 2012; Louw et al., 2016).

## 2.3 The temporomandibular joint (TMJ)

### 2.3.1 Anatomy

Lomas et al (2018) describes the temporomandibular joint as a ginglymoarthrodial joint formed by the mandibular condyle fitting into the glenoid fossa of the temporal bone. It is a complex synovial system with two joints separated by an articular disc. This joint is the most frequently used in the body (Ferreira et al., 2016) and enables important movements such as chewing, swallowing and speaking.

The main muscles that play a role in CMD include the masseter muscle, the temporalis muscle and the pterygoid muscles (medial and lateral). The sensory supply to the temporomandibular joint is provided by branches of the trigeminal nerve, in particular the auriculotemporal nerve and the masseteric nerve. The auriculotemporal nerve supplies the temporal region, the outer ear and the eardrum and is particularly sensitive to pain stimuli (Rodriguez-Lopez et al., 2015). The temporomandibular joint is susceptible to functional or pathological changes that can lead to conditions such as CMD (Donnarumma et al., 2010).

### 2.3.2 The joint surfaces

According to de Oliveira et al. (2023, cited in Alomar et al., 2007; Sommer et al., 2003), the temporomandibular joint consists of two bony parts: the temporal component and the mandibular condyle. Both parts are each surrounded by a synovial capsule. The temporal component comprises the squamous epithelium of the temporal bone, the anterior edge of which forms the articular eminence. The mandibular condyle, which protrudes into the joint cavity, has an oval or rounded shape.

### 2.3.3 Musculature

According to Bordoni and Varacallo (2023), the musculature of the temporomandibular joint is crucial for its movement and protection. Closing the jaw is made possible by the masseter, temporalis and pterygoideus lateralis muscles. The pterygoideus medialis, geniohyoideus, mylohyoideus and digastricus muscles are responsible for opening the jaw.

### 2.3.4 Ligamentous apparatus

According to Bordoni and Varacallo (2023), the ligamentous apparatus of the temporomandibular joint regulates forces and transmits proprioceptive signals. The most important ligaments include the sphenomandibular, stylomandibular, pterygomandibular and pinto- or malleolomandibular ligaments. The collateral ligament consists of two symmetrical fibre bundles.

### 2.3.5 Blood supply

According to Bordoni and Varacallo (cited in Cuccia et al., 2013), the temporomandibular joint is supplied with blood mainly via the superficial temporal artery, the maxillary artery and the masseteric artery. Other contributing arterial branches are the posterior auricular artery, the ascending pharyngeal artery and the ascending palatine artery, all of which originate from the external carotid artery. Venous drainage is provided via the pterygoid plexus in the retrodiscal region and includes connections to several veins, including the internal maxillary vein, sphenopalatine vein, middle meningeal vein, profunda temporalis vein, masseteric vein and inferior alveolar vein.

### 2.3.6 Innervation

According to Bordoni and Varacallo (2023, cited in Asaki et al., 2006; Davidson et al., 2003), the temporomandibular joint contains several proprioceptive receptors, such as Golgi-Mazzoni and Ruffini receptors, as well as myelinated and non-myelinated nerve fibres, which are mainly located in the tissue of the articular disc. The joint capsule is innervated in the anterolateral area by the masseteric nerve, a branch of the second branch of the trigeminal nerve. The lateral area of the capsule, on the other hand, is supplied by the auriculotemporal nerve, a branch of the third branch of the trigeminal nerve (cranial nerve V).

### 2.3.7 Discus articularis

According to Bordoni and Varacallo (2023), the articular disc, which lies between the condyle and the glenoid fossa, has a biconcave or oval shape. It is about 2 mm thick at the front and about 3 mm thick at the back, with the centre being thinner. The anterior part consists of an elastic and fibrous layer. At the top, the disc is connected to the postglenoid process, which prevents it from slipping when the mouth is opened. At the bottom, it limits excessive rotational movements in relation to the condyle.

Anteriorly, the articular disc is connected to the joint capsule, the articular eminence, the condyle and the upper part of the lateral pterygoid muscle. Posteriorly, it is connected to the retro-vertebral disc tissue, the glenoid fossa, the condyle and the temporal bone. The medial and lateral surfaces of the disc are attached to the condylar formation of the mandible, while the edges are partially fused to the joint capsule.

### 2.3.8 Bilaminar zone

According to de Oliveira et al. (2023, cited in Tamimi et al., 2018; Salamon & Casselman, 2020; Tamimi et al., 2019), the bilaminar zone, also known as retrodiscal tissue, stabilises the posterior aspect of the TMJ disc and supports the posterior ligament of the disc. This zone consists of two layers: The upper layer (temporal lamina) attaches to the anterior contour of the external auditory canal, while the lower layer attaches to the posterior contour of the mandibular condyle. Between the layers there is elastic tissue with vessels and nerves. The bilaminar zone prevents slippage or excessive rotation of the articular disc when the mouth is opened. In addition, there is a small anterior lamina that extends towards the joint eminence and the mandibular head.

2.3.9 The occlusion

According to Xiong et al. (2023, cited in de Kanter et al., 2018), occlusion plays a central role for the temporomandibular joint in dental research. Clinically, the term "occlusion" encompasses not only the contact or close contact of the teeth in static positions, but also the "dynamic interactions between all elements of the stomatognathic system, such as teeth, supporting tissue, neuromuscular system, bone and temporomandibular joint" (Trup et al., 2008).

For about 100 years, dental occlusion has been considered an important part of CMD treatment (Kandasamy & Greene, 2020). However, since the 1990s, clinical studies and reviews have increasingly emphasised the relevance of the biopsychosocial model in CMDs. These recommend that dentists de-emphasise occlusal characteristics as causative factors for CMDs (Trup et al, 2008; Kandasamy & Greene, 2020; Manfredini et al, 2017; Suvinen et al, 2005). According to Xiong et al., the relationship between CMDs and occlusion remains a controversial topic.

## 2.4 The cervical spine (cervical spine)

According to Wagner (2022), the cervical spine should not be regarded as a uniform system. It can be subdivided into the craniovertebral joints (from the occiput to C3) and the lower cervical spine (C3 to C7). This differentiation is reflected in the morphology and joint mechanics as well as in the muscle dynamics and neurophysiology (Neuhuber, 2005). A detailed overview of the anatomy and biomechanics of the cervical spine can be found in Table 1.

Table 1: Anatomy and biomechanics of the cervical spine, (own illustration 2024), taken from the study by Wagner (2022)

| Segment | ROM | Seg-men t nerve | Important peripheral nerves | Sensitive/sensory characteristics, dermatomes | Motor R. dorsalis | Reflex muscles/ conditions |
|---|---|---|---|---|---|---|
| C0/C1 | Ink/ Rek 24-30 R pass:<5 | C1 | Suboccipitalis, Ansa cervicalis, regionally important | Dura mater in the area of the foramen magnum. (Afferents | - | Short neck muscles: rectus capitis maj.et min, obliquus |
| | SN:5-10 | | Neuroforamina of the brain base v.HN IX-XII | often via anastomosis to 02-N.occ Major) | | capitis sup.et inf |
| 01/02 | R:38-43/ Page SN: ~6 F/E:22 | 02 | Occipitalis major (with 03), Ansa cervicalis | Occipital region, dorsal cranial fossa | ATM (IP/Ins) | - |
| C2/C3 | F/E: 8-12 SN:10/page R:9/page | C3 | Occipitalis minor, Ansa cervicalis, occipital, ctertius, phrenicus | Neck region, facets C2-C4, C3/C4 (transition segment between upper cervical spine / lower cervical spine) | ATM (IP/Ins) | Diaphragm |
| C3/C4 | F/E: 1217 SN:11/ | 04 | Phrenicus (brachial | Facets C3-C5 "scarf" - | ATM (IP/Ins) | Zerchfell (trapezius |

| | | | | | | |
|---|---|---|---|---|---|---|
| | page R: 10/ page | | plexus) | dermatome | | reflex x |
| C4/C5 | Like C3/C4 | 05 | Pl ex. Brachialis, radialis(C5-Th1), musculocutan. (C5-7), axillaris (C56), phrenic. | No trunk dermatoma, shoulder (deltoid muscle) | ATM (IP/Ins) | Diaphragm, deltoid muscle, biceps brachii muscle (biceps reflex) |
| C5/C6 | F/E: 17 21 SN:8/ Page R:10/ Page | C6 | Plex. brachialis, radialis(C5-Th1) .musculocutan. (C5-7), axillaris (056), median. (C6-Th1) | No trunk dermatoma, radial forearm thumb | ATM (IP/Ins) | M.biceps brachii (biceps reflex), M. brachio-radialis |
| C6/C7 | F/E: 16 21 SN: 7/ Page R: 9/Page | 07 | Plex. Brachialis.radialis (05-Th1) .musculocutan. (C5-7), medianus (C6-Th1) | No torso derm forearm up to Dig. II-IV | ATM (IP/Ins) | M.triceps brachii Triceps reflex M.pectural maj. M.pronator teres |
| C7/ Th1 | F/E:9 SN:4/ Page R: 8/page | C8 | Plex. brachialis radialis(C5-th1), medianus (C6-Th1), ulnaris (C8-Th1) | No Rupmfderm forearm Dig. V | ATM (IP/Ins) | Little finger ball muscle, Trömner reflex |
| Th1/ Th2 | F/E:4 SN: 5/ Page R: 9/page | Th1 | Plex. Brachialis radialis (C5-Th1),medianus (C6-Th1), ulnaris (C8-Th1) | None Hull derm ulnar-sided forearm and elbow, symp. Border cord (Horner syndrome | ATM Intercostal - musculatur | M.flexor carpi ulnaris, Hypothenar |

R: rotation, F: flexion, E: extension, Inc: inclination, Rek: reclination, SN: lateral tilt, pas: passive, akt: active, ATM: autochthonous musculature, IP: Irritation points, Ins: Insertion points, ROM: "range of motion, HN: cranial nerve (mod. after Böhni et al., 2015; Hülse et al., 2005; Bogduk & Mercer, 2000; Böhni, 2014; Schünke et al., 2006).

### 2.4.1 The upper cervical spine

Böhni (2014) describes the upper cervical spine as consisting of the occiput (C0), the atlas (C1) and the axis (C2). Neuroanatomically, functionally and clinically, the C2/3 segment is also assigned to the upper cervical spine, as the typical complaints in this region are caused by the cervicotrigeminal convergence at the spinal trigeminal nucleus. This convergence affects the afferents of the C1-3 nerve roots, the trigeminal nerve and other cranial nerves.

Böhni emphasises that the segments C0/1 (articulationes atlantooccipitales) and C1/2 (articulationes atlantoaxiales laterales, atlantodental joint) anatomically form the craniocervical junction (CCJ). Functionally and neuroanatomically, the segments C0/1, C1/2 and C2/3 are also part of the CCJ, as they have a common afferent projection to the nucleus spinalis nervi trigemini.

2.4.1.1 Anatomy and biomechanics of the upper cervical joints

Böhni (2014) describes the upper head joints, the articulationes atlantooccipitales (C0/1), as oval-shaped ball-and-socket joints. The longitudinal oval, convex articular surfaces of the occipital condyles are connected to the concave facies articulares superiores of the atlas. This anatomical arrangement allows the skull to be viewed as a sphere that is supported by the two concave articular surfaces of the atlas. This enables the movements described below:

□ Flexion/extension-roll-slide movement in the transverse axis (X-axis): These movements are bilaterally coupled and represent a physiologically active movement (pitching movement) that is controlled by the suboccipital musculature and is mainly limited by bony structures (Bogduk, 2000). As this movement is segmentally isolated and functional, it is referred to in the manual medical literature as inclination/reclination, in contrast to flexion of the subsequent section of the cervical spine. As a rule, inclination and reclination of 24-30° are possible (Gutmann, 1984).

□ Lateral flexion sliding movement in the sagittal axis (Y-axis): Due to the bilateral coupling, this is predominantly a sliding movement, which is also referred to as "condylar sliding" on the atlas, i.e. a passive accompanying movement during lateral flexion of the head (Dvorák & Grob 2010). It is 5-10° on one side.

□ Rotation - axial rotational movement (Z-axis): Although this is possible, due to the coupling on both sides it can only take place in the sense of an end-degree passive accompanying movement (< 10°).

Böhni (2014) investigated the movement patterns of the upper cervical spine and described the complex processes involved in lateral tilt and rotation in the cervico-occipital transition. When the cervical spine is tilted to the side, the articular surfaces of the occipital condyles move passively in joint C0/1. However, isolated movement in this area alone is not possible, as the lateral tilt is always associated with movements in segments C1/2 and the vertebrae below. This mechanism is known as condylar gliding.

On the side of the inclination, the occiput slides downwards so that the transverse process of the atlas (C1) approaches the palpating finger on the mastoid. At the same time, the lateral tilt in C1/2 leads to a rotation of the atlas to the same side (ipsilateral). This coordinated movement ensures that the upper cervical joints work together harmoniously (Böhni, 2014).

According to Dvorák and Grob (2010), the lateral tilt of the cervical spine causes the atlas to be displaced laterally towards the tilted side. On functional radiographs, this can be seen as an increased distance between the dens and the lateral massa of the atlas. This movement is controlled and stabilised by the contralateral alar ligament.

Böhni (2014) describes that the cranial articular surfaces of the axis (facies articulares superiores), which lie ventrally next to the dens, have a convex shape. The dens has an anterior articular facies that is in contact with the anterior arch of the atlas. The processus articularis inferior, which forms the facet joint C2/3, is located caudally under the anterior parts of the arch. According to Böhni (2014), the axis acts as a "control vertebra" that ensures the even segmental structure of the lower cervical spine.

2.4.1.2 Ligaments of the upper cervical spine

According to Böhni et al. (2014, cited after Dvorák & Grob, 2010, and Dvorák et al., 1988), the transverse ligament of the atlantis extends from the inside of the lateral mass on one side to the other and lies behind the dens axis. It stabilises the dens in the atlantoaxial segment by preventing dorsal displacement. With an average width of 10 mm and a thickness of 2 mm, this ligament plays a central role in stabilising the anterior arch of the atlas. According to Dvorák et al. (1988) and Bogduk (2000), insufficiency of the ligament, such as occurs in rheumatoid polyarthritis, can lead to instability between the atlas and axis. The rotation of segments C1 and C2 is stabilised by the transverse ligament, as explained by Böhni et al. (2014, cited in Dvorák & Grob, 2010; Dvorák et al., 1988). The ligg. alaria limit the axial rotation of the atlas around the axis. As long as these ligaments are intact, no dislocation of the atlas occurs. They fix the head to the dens axis and thus indirectly stabilise the atlas.

Rotation to the left causes the left alar ligament to become tense. As the rotation progresses, the ligament wraps around the dens, which leads to a lateral displacement of the occiput. This mechanism causes a forced lateral tilt of the occiput and the axis until the right ligament is also tensed and the movement stops. This explains the forced left rotation of the axis during lateral flexion to the left (Dvorák & Grob, 2010; Werne, 1957 in Böhni et al., 2014).

2.4.2 The lower cervical spine

According to Böhni et al. (2020), the lower cervical spine comprises the area from C3/C4 to C7/Th1. This section consists of similarly structured cervical vertebral bodies that enable a comparable range of movement in all three dimensions. According to Böhni et al., the Fryett rule, which describes the coupling of movements, applies to the cervical spine from segment C2/3 onwards: If there is a lateral tilt to the right, the cervical vertebral bodies also rotate to the right. This can be seen, for example, in the palpable deviation of the spinous processes to the left. According to Böhni et al., this movement coupling is utilised in manual medicine by combining rotation and contralateral lateral tilt, a technique known as the 15°/15° rule. This method helps to bring the cervical spine into a functional neutral position and protects the vertebral artery during certain manipulative and mobilising procedures.

## 2.5 Neurodynamic connection between the masticatory apparatus and the cervical spine

Da Silva et al. (2023, cited after Ginszt et al., 2022) report that there is a well-documented link between the cervical spine and the temporomandibular joint, although further studies are needed to better understand the pathophysiology of CMD and somatosensory tinnitus . According to Da Silva et al., asymmetry in the activity of the masticatory muscles could be caused by active myofascial trigger points in the trapezius muscle. This suggests that myofascial pain in the neck muscles can influence disorders of the stomatognathic system.

Da Silva et al. (2023, cited in Levine et al., 2007, and Shore et al., 2007) explain that somatosensory stimuli from the upper cervical spine and temporomandibular joint can reach the somatosensory nucleus of the brainstem and transmit signals to the dorsal cochlear nucleus (CN). Disinhibition of the dorsal CN via these pathways could trigger increased neuronal activity in the auditory system, which could cause somatosensory tinnitus. This theory is supported by studies showing that trigger points in the masticatory, neck and shoulder muscles and increased activity in the muscles supplied by the trigeminal nerve can increase tinnitus intensity (Da Silva et al., 2023, cited in Rocha & Sanchez, 2012).

Gil-Martinez et al. (2018, cited after Kaji et al., 1991) explain that the trigeminal nerve has a mixed function and fulfils sensory, motor and autonomic tasks. With its three main branches - the ophthalmic nerve (V1), the maxillary nerve (V2) and the mandibular nerve (V3) - it supplies large parts of the skull and face. According to Bathla and Hegde (2013), the posterior cranial region, the mandibular angle, parts of the external auditory canal and the pharynx are excluded.

## 2.6 Tinnitus

2.6.1 Definition of terms

Langguth et al. (2019, cited in Möller, 2007) describe tinnitus, often referred to as ringing in the ears, as a widespread disorder that is divided into objective and subjective forms. In objective tinnitus, sufferers perceive sounds that can also be observed by others, for example through turbulent blood flow or muscle contractions. According to Langguth et al., subjective tinnitus, which occurs in most people, is much more common. It is defined as the perception of sounds for which there is neither an external nor an internal sound source (Langguth et al., 2019, quoted from Möller, 2007, and Jastreboff, 1990).

### 2.6.2 Pathophysiology

According to Michiels (2023, cited in van Dijk, 2016), the pathophysiology of tinnitus is often associated with peripheral hearing loss. This can affect hearing or manifest itself as a "hidden hearing loss", in which sound processing is impaired above the hearing threshold. Despite this link, the brain is thought to play a central role in the pathophysiology of tinnitus (Michiels, 2023, cited in Elgoyhen et al., 2015). One model of subjective tinnitus hypothesises that connections in the brainstem between somatosensory and auditory nuclei may influence how somatosensory stimuli alter the loudness and pitch of existing tinnitus or cause it (Michiels, 2023, cited in Levine, 1999). Numerous studies in humans and animals have since demonstrated the involvement of cortical networks in the development and modulation of tinnitus (Michiels, 2023).

### 2.6.3 Causes and risk factors

In their recent study, Tsang et al. (2024) identified various causes, risk factors and concomitant diseases for tinnitus:

□ Hearing loss and cochlear damage: Age and hearing loss are among the main risk factors (Biswas et al., 2022; Lewkowski et al., 2022). Loud noises in particular, which damage the cochlea, are often associated with tinnitus. Other causes include diseases such as blocked ears, middle ear infections, otosclerosis and Meniere's disease.

□ Neurological and vascular causes: Diseases that affect the auditory pathway, such as vestibular schwannoma, migraines and concussions, can trigger tinnitus. Patients with tinnitus and headaches are often particularly affected (Michiels et al., 2018; Langguth et al., 2017).

□ Somatosensory causes: Changes in sensory perception, for example due to problems with the cervical spine or temporomandibular joint, can trigger or exacerbate tinnitus. Typical symptoms include teeth grinding, stress-related jaw clenching, headaches, dizziness, neck pain and temporomandibular joint problems (Langguth et al., 2017).

Hyperacusis: This abnormal intolerance to everyday sounds often leads to physical discomfort. People with tinnitus often report that loud noises can make their tinnitus worse (Westcott, 2009), which can lead to hyperacusis. Around 50 % of tinnitus sufferers also suffer from hyperacusis (Westcott, 2013; Schecklmann et al., 2014).

Psychological and psychiatric comorbidities: Research and clinical experience show a bidirectional relationship between stress, anxiety, depression and fatigue on the one hand and the intensity and severity of tinnitus on the other. These factors also influence the ability to spontaneously habituate to tinnitus (Park et al., 2022; Weber et al., 2022; Han et al., 2018).

□ Environmental factors: In Australia, tinnitus has been shown to be more common in people exposed to hazardous noise levels, such as car workers, drivers and farmers (Lewkowski et al., 2022). Professional musicians are particularly affected, with a prevalence of 26%, which is significantly higher than in the general population (Di Stadio et al., 2018).

### 2.6.4 Classification

According to Oostendorp et al. (2016, cited after Zenner, 1998), the classification of tinnitus begins with the distinction between objective and subjective tinnitus. Objective tinnitus can be heard by both the person affected and the examiner, while subjective tinnitus is only perceived by the person affected. Subjective tinnitus is the most common form and cannot be measured objectively. Various mechanisms that can lead to subjective tinnitus have been described in the literature (Zenner, 1998; Shore et al., 2007; Baguley et al., 2013; Levine & Oron, 2015).

Within subjective tinnitus, a further subdivision is made in which peripheral tinnitus is related to the anatomical region of the ear, i.e. the outer, middle or inner ear, and can be subdivided into conductive and sensorineural tinnitus. Central tinnitus is divided into primary and secondary central tinnitus. Primary central tinnitus originates directly in the brain, while secondary central tinnitus or tinnitus sensitisation describes a condition in which peripherally triggered tinnitus manifests itself independently of its source in the brain. Oostendorp et al. summarise the classification by categorising the main types of tinnitus according to their anatomical and functional origin (Zenner, 1998). In the literature, the main types of tinnitus are categorised as follows:

2.6.4.1 Objective tinnitus

According to Fobbe et al. (2022), objective tinnitus is caused by an endogenous sound source, such as vascular anomalies of the carotid artery, and can be detected by listening.

2.6.4.2 Subjective tinnitus

According to Fobbe et al. (2022, cited in Mazurek et al., 2017), subjective tinnitus occurs more frequently than objective tinnitus. The cause is usually suspected to be in the inner ear or in suboptimal processing of auditory information, often accompanied by hearing loss. The exact central mechanisms are not yet fully understood. If the ringing in the ears does not affect those affected, it is referred to as compensated tinnitus, which is categorised as grade 1 (no discomfort) and grade 2 (occurring in silence and disturbing under stress or strain). In contrast, a level of distress indicates decompensated tinnitus, which can lead to permanent private or professional impairment (grade 3) or to complete decompensation and occupational disability (grade 4). In addition, decompensated tinnitus can lead to comorbidities such as depressive episodes or anxiety disorders.

2.6.4.3 Somatosensory tinnitus

According to Michiels et al. (2018), somatosensory tinnitus is a subtype of subjective tinnitus in which altered somatosensory signals from the cervical spine or temporomandibular joint influence or trigger the perception of tinnitus. As early as the 1990s, researchers such as Hiller, Janca and Burke (1997) and Pinchoff et al. (1998) investigated the influence of the somatosensory system on tinnitus complaints. In 1999, Levine presented the hypothesis of a tinnitus subtype for the first time, which he called "somatic tinnitus".

Sharma et al. (2021, cited after Michiels et al., 2018) describe somatic or somatosensory tinnitus as a result of diseases of the cervical spine or the temporo-mandibular region. These can modulate the volume and pitch of the tinnitus. The prevalence of somatic tinnitus is around 36-43% in the Belgian population, with cervicogenic tinnitus occurring in 43% and temporomandibular disorders in 64% of those affected (Sharma et al., 2021, cited in Michiels et al., 2018; Sajadi et al., 2019). Such disorders are also common in patients with dental pulpitis (Sharma et al., 2021, cited in Niedrig et al., 2017).

Haider et al (2017) list various signs of somatosensory tinnitus, including head and neck problems such as TMJ syndrome, osteophytes, osteoarthritis, spondylosis, myofascial trigger points and dental or jaw disease. Frequent pain in the head, neck or shoulder area, poor posture, bruxism and a worsening of symptoms with the simultaneous occurrence of pain and tinnitus are also typical characteristics (Sanchez & Rocha, 2011b, c). Due to these complex symptoms, a multidisciplinary team of dentists and physiotherapists is often necessary to ensure a precise diagnosis and treatment.

CMD-associated tinnitus

According to Bousema et al. (2018), numerous studies show a close connection between tinnitus and CMD. This relationship is bidirectional: people with tinnitus have an increased risk of developing CMD, while CMD patients are also more likely to have tinnitus. Although most studies confirm this relationship, none of the studies analysed were of high quality. Weaknesses such as lack of blinding or lack of comparability of the groups increased the risk of biased results.

Bousema et al. (2018) also report that almost all studies found an unspecific link between CMD and tinnitus. One exception is the study by De Felicio et al. (2008), which provides more specific findings. One study compared CMD in patients with and without tinnitus (Park & Moon, 2014), while five other studies analysed tinnitus in CMD patients (Buergers et al, 2014; De Felicio et al, 1999; De Felicio et al, 2008; Effat, 2016; Fernandes et al, 2013).

Overall, 37-88% of CMD patients from specialised clinics reported tinnitus. The weighted odds ratios ranged from 1.7 to 44.3, with an overall odds ratio of 6.7 (95% CI) (Akhter et al., 2013; Baguley et al., 2002; Dworkin & LeResche, 1992; Bornstein et al., 2009). According to Bousema et al., CMD can be arthrogenic (CMDa) or myogenic (CMDm). In CMDa, eight out of eleven studies showed a connection with tinnitus. The frequency of tinnitus in CMD patients from specialised clinics was between 20% and 59%, while it was between 21% and 48% in other patient groups. Eight studies investigated CMDa in patients with and without tinnitus (Bernhardt et al, 2004; Camparis et al, 2005; Hilgenberg et al, 2012; Khedr et al, 2010; Kuttila et al, 2005; Peroz, 2003; Pezzoli et al, 2015; Rubinstein, 1993), and three studies analysed tinnitus in CMDa patients (Akhter et al, 2013; Parker & Chole, 1995; Tuz et al, 2003). The odds ratios ranged from 1.2 to 9.9, with an overall odds ratio of 2.3 (95% CI) (Abel & Levine, 2004; Bernhardt et al, 2004; Baguley et al, 2013; Bjorne, 2007).

In the case of CMDm, all seven studies found a significant correlation with tinnitus. These studies focussed on myofascial pain in the jaw area. Five studies investigated CMDm in patients with and without tinnitus (Bernhardt et al, 2004; Camparis et al, 2005; Hilgenberg et al, 2012; Leher et al, 2003; Pezzoli et al, 2015), while one study analysed tinnitus in CMDm patients (Tuz et al, 2003). The odds ratios ranged from 1.3 to 10.0, with an overall odds ratio of 4.1 (95% CI) (Akhter et al., 2013; Abel & Levine, 2004; Borenstein et al., 2009).

Cervicogenic somatosensory tinnitus (CST)

Michiels et al (2016, citing Pfaller and Arvidsson, 1988; Zhan, 2006) describe CST as a form of tinnitus related to the cervical spine and its somatic system. Animal studies show that there is a connection between the cervical somatosensory system and the CN, which provides the physiological basis for CST. According to Shore et al (2007), somatosensory information from the cervical spine is transmitted to the brain via afferent fibres. These fibres have their cell bodies in the spinal ganglia or in the trigeminal ganglion and also partially project into the central auditory system. There they influence the firing rate or synchrony of the neurones and can thus change the intensity and characteristics of the tinnitus. Shore et al. (2007) as well as Young et al. (1995), Kanold and Young (2001), Zhan et al. (2006), Shore et al. (2008) and Shore (2011) confirm neural connections between the auditory system and the cervical spine through animal studies. This concept is based on the convergence of auditory signals from the cochlea and somatosensory input from the face and the cervical structures (C1-C4) at the CN. The somatosensory neurones in the dorsal CN and in the caudal part of the spinal tract of the trigeminal nerve (V) are particularly affected. According to Nieuwenhuys et al (1988), there are additional connections to the outer and middle ear via the common spinal tract of the cranial nerves (VII, IX and X). Many of these ascending pathways from the CN ultimately project to the auditory cortex. A schematic model hypothesising the dorsal CN in the context of CST is described by Levine et al. (2007, cited in Levine and Oron, 2015). According to this model, prolonged noxious activity, such as whiplash or chronic neck pain, can disinhibit dorsal CN and exacerbate tinnitus. These connections are shown schematically in Figure 1.

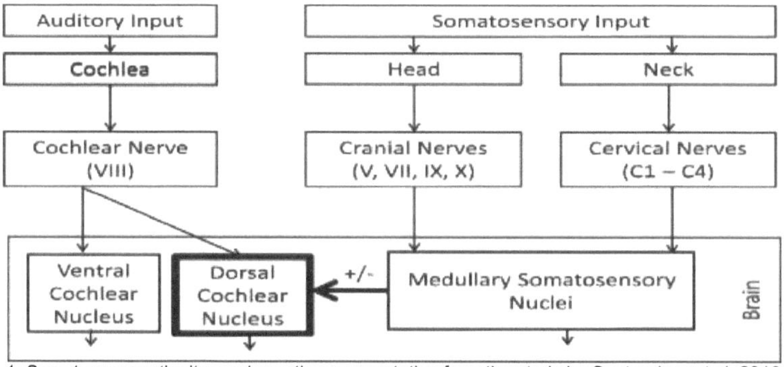

Figure 1: Somatosensory tinnitus, schematic representation from the study by Oostendrop et al, 2016 cited from Levine et al, 2007 Levine and Oron, 2015.

Figure 1: Schematic representation of the anatomical and physiological basis for the modulation of somatosensory tinnitus. **+** = Disinhibition of the somatosensory subgroup of the dorsal cochlear nucleus (increased tinnitus). - = Inhibition of the somatosensory subgroup of the dorsal cochlear nucleus (reduced tinnitus). **V** = trigeminal nerve; **VII** = facial nerve; **VIII** = cochlear nerve; **IX** = glossopharyngeal nerve; **X** = vagus nerve. **C1-C4** = cervical spinal nerves

2.6.4.4 Pulsatile tinnitus

Langguth et al. (2024, cited in De Ridder, 2011, and De Ridder et al., 2007) report that pulsatile, pulse-synchronised tinnitus can indicate an abnormality in blood flow. Possible causes are vascular anomalies such as stenoses, arteriovenous fistulas or malformations. Increased blood flow, for example in anaemia, could also play a role. More rarely, a microvascular conflict is the cause.

Langguth et al. explain that many patients with pulse-synchronised tinnitus show no obvious vascular abnormalities. One possible explanation for this is an increased sensitivity to body sounds. Those affected perceive sounds that are generated by blood flow and transmitted to the inner ear via bone conduction. In addition, increased intracranial pressure could intensify this transmission (cited in Sismanis, 1998).

2.6.4.5 Psychosomatic tinnitus

Langguth et al. (2024, cited after Elarbed et al., 2021, and Patil et al., 2023) report that many patients state that their tinnitus becomes more intense in stressful situations. This could be explained by an increased alertness to sensory signals under sympathetic activation. However, not all people react to stress in the same way. Patil et al. (2023) show that stress can influence both the development and worsening of tinnitus. They suggest that future studies should combine auditory and emotional systems to better understand the link between stress and tinnitus. Such research could help to prevent stress-induced tinnitus and more accurately assess the prognosis for patients.

According to Herbert et al. (2012), depression is also considered a risk factor for tinnitus, especially if it is accompanied by additional symptoms. Patel et al. (2020) show in a meta-analysis that the prevalence of depression in patients with Meniere's disease is "close to an astonishing 50%". Tinnitus is also associated with anxiety disorders (Pattyn et al., 2016).

These findings suggest that tinnitus, anxiety and depression may utilise shared brain networks. Alternatively, tinnitus and accompanying symptoms could promote the activation of depression networks (De Ridder et al., 2014; Langguth et al., 2011, 2023; Pattyn et al., 2018).

2.6.5 Localisation

According to Langguth et al. (2024, cited after Shin et al., 2023), tinnitus is perceived differently: unilateral (approx. 45 %), bilateral (approx. 45 %) or non-lateralised (approx. 10 %). This variability can be partially explained by unilateral hearing loss, as tinnitus often occurs on the side of the hearing loss, which supports the deafferentation theory. However, it remains unclear which factors influence the exact localisation of tinnitus, especially in patients who perceive it in the head.

Langguth et al. also report that some patients have difficulty localising their tinnitus precisely or state that the localisation changes over time. Studies also show that the perceived pitch of tinnitus often coincides with the area of most severe hearing loss (Norena et al., 2002; Schecklmann et al., 2012). This supports the theory that tinnitus arises as a phantom sound that is triggered by the brain's attempt to compensate for a lack of auditory input (Jastreboff, 1990).

These findings suggest that tinnitus may be caused by inadequate feed-forward inhibition. According to Roberts et al. (2008, cited in Langguth et al., 2024), a lack of lateral inhibition could result in a tinnitus pitch in the range between normal hearing and hearing loss.

### 2.6.6 Diagnostics

According to Dalrymple et al (2021), the main goal of medical care for patients with tinnitus should be to identify causes that are either treatable or potentially dangerous. A targeted history and physical examination are the most important tools for differentiating between benign and serious causes and choosing appropriate treatment options.

Dalrymple et al. emphasise that the initial triage should identify features that require urgent investigation. These include, for example, pulsatile tinnitus associated with neurological symptoms, unilateral discomfort, asymmetrical hearing loss or other abnormalities. According to Hofmann et al. (2013), pulsatile tinnitus, although less common, may indicate cardiovascular disease, intracranial vascular abnormalities, increased intracranial pressure or neoplasia.

Dalrymple et al. name four central elements of the medical history for the assessment of tinnitus: chronicity, localisation (unilateral or bilateral), associated hearing changes and the effects (disturbing or not disturbing).

If MRI is not available or there are contraindications for contrast agents, alternatives such as non-contrast MRI, auditory brainstem response test or CT are available. According to Fortnum et al (2009), non-contrast MRI has a similar sensitivity to conventional MRI for vestibular schwannomas, but is less suitable for detecting other causes. Auditory brainstem response testing is reliable for lesions larger than 1 cm, but less so for smaller lesions. CT can reveal vascular or bony lesions but miss small masses (Kessler et al., 2017).

According to Dalrymple et al., laboratory tests are only useful if there is a clinical suspicion of specific underlying diseases. Earlier studies that suspected links between tinnitus and diseases such as thyroid problems, vitamin B12 deficiency or diabetes are based on low-quality evidence. According to Shargorodsky et al. (2010), Kazmierczak and Doroszewska (2001), Klagenberg et al. (2007), Sutbas et al. (2007) and Cochran and Kosmicki (1979), routine testing for these conditions is not justified.

### 2.6.7 Therapeutic approaches

Langguth et al. (2024) emphasise the heterogeneity of tinnitus with regard to the response to treatment. Many of the therapeutic approaches investigated showed no significant difference between the intervention and control groups and were therefore rated as less successful. However, the response varied greatly: some participants responded positively to the therapy, while the majority showed no or even a negative response (Langguth et al., 2024). The European Multidisciplinary Guideline for Tinnitus recommends various treatment options, including cochlear implants, hearing aids, neurostimulation, cognitive behavioural therapy, pharmacotherapy, tinnitus retraining therapy, sound therapy (e.g. maskers), as well as dietary and alternative approaches such as acupuncture. Of these, only cognitive behavioural therapy shows a high level of evidence for its effectiveness in tinnitus and is therefore strongly recommended. Pharmacotherapy is not directly effective against tinnitus, but can alleviate tinnitus-associated disorders such as depression or stress (Fobbe et al., 2022, cited in Cima et al., 2019).

Physiotherapy treatment: Van der Wal et al. (2020) suggested conservative orofacial therapy for patients with somatosensory tinnitus caused by CMD. This multimodal intervention includes counselling, stretching exercises, massages of the masticatory muscles and relaxation therapy. In some cases, a bite splint was also recommended. For patients with additional cervical spine problems, cervical spine mobilisation and targeted exercises were integrated (Da Silva et al., 2023, cited in Van der Wal et al., 2020).

In their study, Oostendorp et al (2016) refer to several papers that identified a neural connection between the dorsal cochlear nucleus and the somatosensory systems of the head and upper cervical spine as a possible cause of tinnitus in patients with cervicogenic somatosensory tinnitus. A broader understanding of (chronic) somatosensory tinnitus could help to establish manual therapy as a proven method for the assessment and treatment of patients with cervicogenic somatosensory tinnitus.

In their study, Michiels et al. (2018) reported new findings on the significant improvement of tinnitus through TENS (Herraiz et al., 2007; Vanneste et al., 2010). TENS in skin areas near the ear promotes activation of the dorsal cochlear nucleus via the somatosensory pathway. This may enhance the inhibitory role of this nucleus in the central nervous system and thereby alleviate tinnitus (Herraiz et al., 2007). Herraiz et al. (2007, cited in Michiels et al., 2018) showed that TENS led to improvement in 46% of patients with somatic tinnitus after two weeks, as measured by reduced VAS tinnitus severity scores. They also found that tinnitus caused by somatosensory injury responded better to treatment than somatic tinnitus associated with otological disease.

Chiropractic therapy: Michiels et al (2018) report that chiropractic therapy aims to counteract abnormal movement patterns by manipulating the spine and extremities. Only three studies on chiropractic treatment of tinnitus were found, all based on case studies. Alcantara et al. (2002, cited in Michiels et al., 2018) described the treatment of a 41-year-old female patient suffering from ear pain, tinnitus, dizziness, altered hearing, ear infections and headaches. CMD and cervical subluxations were diagnosed. After nine treatments over two months, the authors reported complete relief of CMD symptoms, including tinnitus. The therapy involved rapid, low-amplitude adjustments.

Kessinger and Boneva (2000, cited in Michiels et al., 2018) reported on a 75-year-old patient who showed improvements in dizziness, tinnitus and hearing loss after chiropractic treatment of the upper cervical spine. The authors attributed the success of the therapy to improved cervical spine function.

□ Drug treatment: Langguth et al. (2019, cited after Cederroth et al., 2013) report that despite the great market potential, there are currently no approved pharmacological treatments for tinnitus. Efforts in industrial research and development also appear to be limited.

Tinnitus retraining therapy (TRT): Tsang et al. (2024, cited by Phillips & McFerran) report that TRT is based on Jastreboff's neurophysiological model and is a widely used treatment method. It combines the principles of this model with low-volume neutral sound stimuli to reduce the intensity of the tinnitus signal. A Cochrane review showed that TRT is significantly more effective than tinnitus masking.

□ Audiological therapy: Tsang et al. (2024) recommend the passive use of broadband sounds at low volume, such as white noise or ocean/rain sounds, for disturbing tinnitus. These sounds can help to create a calming sound environment and reduce awareness of the tinnitus, especially in quiet moments. Various apps for smartphones and tablets offer a wide range of customisable sounds that can be individually adjusted in volume and duration.

- Cognitive behavioural therapy (CBT): Tsang et al. (2024, cited in McKenna et al., 2014) describe that CBT is based on the assumption that negative cognitive misinterpretations of the tinnitus signal and physical arousal lead to incorrect evaluations, distorted perceptions and tinnitus hypervigilance. These processes promote negative thinking and increase stress. A Cochrane review showed that CBT has low to moderate efficacy in reducing the negative impact of tinnitus on patients' quality of life (Tsang et al., 2024, cited in Fuller et al., 2020).
- Hearing aids and cochlear implants: Langguth et al. (2024, cited after Waechter & Jonsson, 2022) report that an improvement in hearing in tinnitus patients with hearing loss can also lead to a reduction in tinnitus. This was observed both with the use of hearing aids and cochlear implants (Langguth et al., 2024, cited in Borges et al., 2021; Yuen et al., 2021). This finding supports the theory that tinnitus can be caused by the brain's efforts to compensate for reduced auditory input. The effect is particularly pronounced with cochlear implants, as these directly stimulate the deafferentated auditory nerve fibres (Langguth et al., 2024, cited in Peter et al., 2019).

Neurofeedback (NFB) therapy: Xiaoyan et al. (2022) describe NFB therapy as a non-invasive, electrophysiological approach that visualises brain activity parameters. This enables patients to specifically change their brain activity and regulate these parameters either positively or negatively.

# CHAPTER 3

# 3 Methodology

## 3.1 Research questions

### 3.1.1 Primary research question

This master's thesis examines the primary research question: "How effective is physiotherapy in the treatment of tinnitus associated with CMD or upper cervical spine?". To answer this question, a systematic review was conducted. This was based on the analysis of ten RCTs identified in a structured and reproducible literature search.

However, the work not only aims to clarify the primary research question, but also to answer secondary questions that can be derived from it. It became apparent that not all secondary questions could be fully answered by the ten selected RCTs. Despite thorough and systematic searches in relevant databases, suitable RCTs were missing for some of these questions. It was therefore necessary to draw on other high-quality studies with different study designs in order to answer the secondary questions in the best possible way and to support the results with verifiable data.

### 3.1.2 Secondary research questions

To comprehensively answer the primary research question, two secondary research questions were formulated to examine specific aspects of the primary question in more detail. These questions relate to the following areas:

#### 3.1.2.1 Connection between CMD and tinnitus

Granada et al. (2016, cited after Bernhardt et al., 2011) report that CMD could act as a predisposing factor for the development of tinnitus. In a study with 3,300 participants, it was found that people with CMD, regardless of factors such as gender, age, education level and frequent headaches, had a 2 to 4-fold increased risk of developing tinnitus within five years. The exact type of CMD most commonly associated with tinnitus remains unclear. Some studies show that tinnitus is more common with intra-articular lesions such as displacement of the temporomandibular joint disc, especially when found on the side of unilateral tinnitus. These lesions often occurred in conjunction with mild orofacial pain (Granada et al., 2016, citing Ren and Isberg, 1995). In contrast, other studies found tinnitus to be more strongly associated with isolated myofascial headaches or TMJ pain than with internal derangements, isolated clicking or restricted mouth opening (Granada et al., 2016, cited in Tullberg & Ernberg, 2006; Akter et al., 2013). However, due to the small sample sizes in previous studies, these differences could not be clearly confirmed statistically (Granada et al., 2016, cited in Akter et al., 2013).

Miyamoto et al. (2024) examined 76 patients between April and May 2023 who took part in an audiometric examination. The average age was 69.7 years (± 12.8), with an age range from 42 to 95 years. It was found that 90.8 % of patients ($n = 69$) were affected by some form of temporomandibular joint disorder. Of these, 46.1 % had mild, 34.2 % had moderate and 10.5 % had severe disease.

42 patients (55.3 %) also suffered from tinnitus. The study showed a significant correlation between temporomandibular joint disorders and tinnitus ($p = 0.022$). In addition, a higher severity of TMJ disorder was associated with a higher probability of tinnitus ($p = 0.043$). The odds ratio (OR) showed that patients with temporomandibular joint disorders had an 8.8-fold increased risk of tinnitus, with the risk increasing 42-fold in the case of severe dysfunction.

Miyamoto et al (2024) also investigated the relationship between tinnitus, temporomandibular joint disorders and other diseases. They found no significant association between tinnitus and hearing loss ($p = 0.879$), hypertension ($p = 0.595$) or migraine ($p = 0.916$). However, there was a significant correlation between temporomandibular joint disorders and tinnitus in patients with hearing loss ($p = 0.046$). No comparable correlations were found for high blood pressure and migraine (p = 0.131 and p = 0.147 respectively). These results confirm that the severity of TMJ disorder correlates strongly with the likelihood of tinnitus and underline the relevance of CMD in the development of tinnitus.

3.1.2.2 Connection between upper cervical spine and tinnitus

Wadhwa et al. (2024, cited in Peng et al., 2015) emphasise that cervical spine abnormalities can impair blood flow to the auditory pathways. Spasm or compression of the vertebral artery can cause transient ischaemia in areas of the brain responsible for auditory processing. This vascular component can exacerbate the symptoms of tinnitus.

Michiels et al. (2015, cited after Abel and Levine, 2004; Fabijanska et al., 2014; Ostermann et al., 2014) report that cervicogenic somatic tinnitus (CST) occurs in around 36-43% of tinnitus sufferers. Patients with CST often show limited mobility of the cervical spine, especially during rotational movements. In addition, combined movements such as extension, lateral tilt and rotation can trigger pain (Michiels et al., 2015, cited in Reisshauer et al., 2006). Sensitive trigger points in the cervical spine are also typical of CST (Michiels et al., 2015, cited in Reisshauer et al., 2006). A high score on the Neck Bournemouth Questionnaire (NBQ), over 14 out of 70 points, is also considered an indication of CST (Michiels et al., 2015, cited in Reisshauer et al., 2006).

These results emphasise the influence of the upper cervical spine on the development and severity of tinnitus.

## 3.2 Search strategy

To answer the primary research question and the derived secondary questions, a systematic literature search was conducted in the MEDLINE (PubMed and PMC), PEDro and ScienceDirect databases. For the primary research question, a targeted search was conducted for RCTs published within the last twelve years. The RCTs had to address the main aspects of the research question, namely physiotherapy, CMD, upper cervical spine and tinnitus. Studies that addressed at least three of these aspects - in particular physiotherapy and tinnitus in combination with CMD or upper cervical spine - were also included. For the secondary research questions investigating the relationship between tinnitus and CMD and between tinnitus and the upper cervical spine, studies of different designs were considered. The aim was to comprehensively illuminate and scientifically substantiate these relationships. In addition, the reference lists of the identified studies were systematically searched in order to find further relevant studies that could be included in the analysis.

## 3.3 PICO scheme

Tab 2: PICO scheme (own illustration 2024)

| | |
|---|---|
| Population | Patients with CMD or upper cervical spine disorders and tinnitus |
| Intervention | Physiotherapy |
| Comparison | Other interventions or placebo |
| Outcome | Relief of CMD or upper cervical spine associated tinnitus |

## 3.4 Inclusion and exclusion criteria

Tab 3: Inclusion and exclusion criteria of the included studies (own presentation 2024)

| Variables | Inclusion criteria | Exclusion criteria |
|---|---|---|
| T ext availability | Full text | Not available in full text |
| Language | No restrictions | - |
| Study design | Randomised controlled trial Studies (RCT) | Other study designs |
| Publication date | 2012-2024 | Before 2012 |
| Population | Patients with tinnitus and at | Patients with tinnitus but without |

| | | |
|---|---|---|
| | least CMD or upper cervical spine disorder | CMD or without upper cervical spine disorder |
| Intervention | Physiotherapy, placebo or other interventions | Studies without physiotherapy |
| Outcome | Tinnitus relief | Not specified |
| Setting | No restriction | - |

### 3.5 Analysis of the evidence classes

The classification defined by the Oxford Centre for Evidence Based Medicine (CEBM) in 2009 (Howick, 2009) is used to interpret the evidence class or the hierarchy level of the strength of evidence. Table 4 below shows the analysis of the evidence classes:

Tab 4: Analysis of the evidence classes (own presentation 2024)

| **Level** | **Description of the** |
|---|---|
| **1 a** | SR (with homogeneous results) of different RCTs |
| **1 b** | RCT with narrow confidence interval |
| **1 c** | "All or none" case series |
| **II a** | SR (with homogeneous results) of different cohort studies |
| **II b** | Cohort studies, methodologically weak RCTs (e.g. follow-up <80%) |
| **II c** | Outcome studies, ecological research |
| **III a** | SR (with homogeneous results) via case-control studies |
| **III b** | Case-control studies |
| **IV** | Case series, methodologically weak cohort and case-control studies |
| **V** | Expert opinions |

### 3.6 Literature sources

3.6.1 **Medline** (PubMed and PMC)

3.6.1.1 Search strategy

During the literature search in the PubMed database, the search period was regularly updated in order to identify as many relevant RCTs as possible. Three weeks before the work was completed, a final review and update was carried out to ensure that all current publications were included.

The last search initially found 101 studies. By using the "Publication Date" filter (2012-2024), 41 studies were excluded. The filter "Text Availability" (only full texts) reduced the number by a further two studies. Finally, the filter "Article Type" (Randomised Controlled Trials) resulted in a final selection of seven studies. Of these seven studies, one was excluded because access to the full text was not possible. A further study was excluded as it did not contain any results and was only accessible to prioritised users. This left five studies that largely answered the primary research question and the research questions.

3.6.1.2 Search terms

Search terms in three main areas were used for the systematic literature search:

Temporomandibular dysfunction**:** Temporomandibular disorder, TMD, temporomandibular dysfunction, CMD, craniomandibular dysfunction, jaw disorder, upper cervical spine, upper cervical vertebrae, cervical spine, cervicocephalic region.

Tinnitus: Tinnitus, ear ringing, ear noise, subjective tinnitus, somatosensory tinnitus, somatic tinnitus, cervical tinnitus, cervicogenic tinnitus, neck related tinnitus.

Physiotherapy: Physiotherapy, physical therapy, manual therapy, manual therapy, physical rehabilitation, therapeutic exercise.

These search terms were specifically combined to identify relevant studies in the areas of CMD, cervical spine, tinnitus and physiotherapy.

3.6.1.3 Filter

The filters "Publication Date" (2012- 2024), "Text Availability" (full texts only) and "Article Type" (Randomised Controlled Trial) were used for the search.

3.6.1.4 Search protocol

The search protocol for the literature search is shown in Fig. 4 in the appendix.

3.6.2 **PEDro** (Physiotherapy Evidence Database)

3.6.2.1 Search strategy

The search in the PEDro database was carried out using the "Advanced Search" function. The following settings were used:

- Field Abstract & Title: CMD, Tinnitus, Physiotherapy
- Field therapy: stretching, mobilisation, manipulation, massage
- Field Problem: no appropriate value in this field
- Field Body Part: head or neck
- Field Subdiscipline: orthopaedics
- Field Topic: no appropriate value in this field
- Field Method: clinical trial
- Field Published Since: 2012

Firstly, the search terms were combined with "Match all search terms" (AND) (see Appendix, Fig. 5). This search yielded no hits ("No records found").

The search was then customised by linking the terms with "Match any search terms" (OR). This resulted in 264,751 hits from various areas (see Appendix, Fig. 6).

An additional "Simple Search" was carried out, which can only combine terms with "OR" (see Appendix, Fig. 7). The search terms "tinnitus" and "somatosensory tinnitus" returned 59 studies.

Of these, one practice guideline and 15 systematic reviews were excluded as they were not RCTs. 43 clinical trials remained for further analysis, of which 6 RCTs were selected as suitable. Three of these RCTs were removed due to duplicates, so that ultimately 3 studies were included in the research.

3.6.2.2 Search terms

Tinnitus, Somatosensory tinnitus

3.6.2.3 Filter

Not selectable

3.6.2.4 Search protocol

The search protocol for the literature search is shown in Fig. 8 in the appendix.

3.6.3 **Science Direct**

3.6.3.1 Search strategy

For literature searches in the ScienceDirect database, the function "Advanced Search" was used. The search screen only offered limited options, as only the fields "Find articles with these terms" and "Years" were relevant for the search (see Appendix, Fig. 9).

Various search combinations were tested, including "tinnitus, physiotherapy, manual therapy, TMD, temporomandibular disorder, CMD, somatosensory tinnitus". However, most of them did not provide any relevant results. The term "somatosensory tinnitus" finally proved to be the most effective and led to 999 hits in the first search (see Appendix, Fig. 10).

For further narrowing down, the filter "Medicine and Dentistry" was applied in the "Subject Areas" section, which reduced the number of hits to 570 studies (see Appendix, Fig. 11).

As ScienceDirect does not offer any further filtering options, such as for RCTs, the 570 studies were screened manually. After this screening, 5 RCTs were identified as suitable. Of these, 3 were excluded due to duplicates, so that 2 RCTs were ultimately included in the research.

3.6.3.2 Search terms
Somatosensory tinnitus
3.6.3.3 Filter
The following filters were used for the search:

- Year(s): 2012-2024
- Subject Areas: Medicine and Dentistry

3.6.3.4 Search protocol
The two search protocols are shown in Figs. 10 and 11 in the appendix.

## 3.7 Selection and evaluation of the studies

The literature research for this master's thesis began around 15 months ago. At the beginning, a broad approach was taken by reviewing literature, specialised articles and journals from different fields in order to create a solid basis. Over time, the research became increasingly precise by introducing targeted search strategies and restrictions in order to work out the relevance of the research questions.
Until shortly before the Master's thesis was completed, the literature research was continuously reviewed, supplemented and revised to ensure a precise presentation. Numerous studies of different designs were analysed, which are listed under the term "secondary studies" in the bibliography. These studies were used to answer the secondary research questions and to shed light on specific aspects of the research questions. Ten RCTs were selected to answer the primary research question. These were taken from three renowned databases:
PEDro: 3 studies
PubMed and PMC: 5 studies
ScienceDirect: 2 studies
The search strategies were customised to the options and properties of the respective databases. Optimised search methods and specific filters were used to increase the efficiency and accuracy of the search.
The focus was on high-quality RCTs that covered the relevant main concepts of the research questions. Suitable assessment tools were used to analyse the selected RCTs, including
PRISMA flow chart
PEDro scale
CONSORT 2010 checklist
Cochrane Risk of Bias Tool (RoB1)
A systematic review of the limitations of the studies
This methodological approach ensures a transparent and high-quality evaluation of the included studies. The results of the analyses are presented in tabular form in order to provide a clear and concise presentation.
3.7.1 PRISMA 2020 flow chart
According to Rethlefsen et al. (2022, cited in Page et al., 2021), the PRISMA 2020 template offers systematic review teams an improved opportunity to detail the complexity of the search process. With this update, not only database searches, but also study registers and other sources can be recorded more precisely. A total of four different templates are available, including specially developed versions for updates and systematic reviews that go beyond databases and trial registries (Page et al., 2021). This further development makes it possible to make the process more transparent and better meet the requirements of modern systematic reviews (Rethlefsen et al., 2022). Fig 2 below provides a PRISMA 2020.

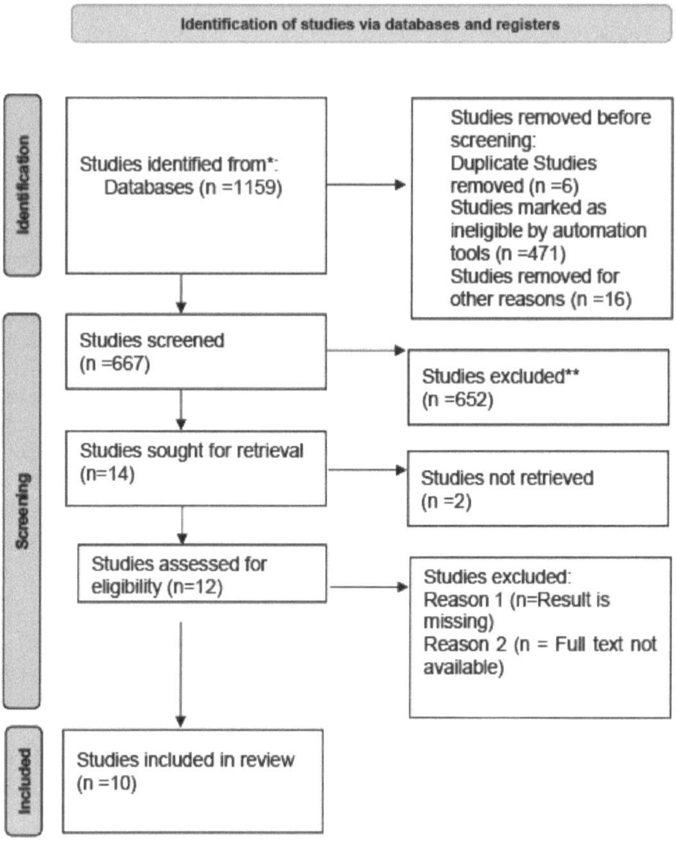


Fig 2: PRISMA 2020 flow chart of the included studies (own illustration 2024)

3.7.2 Assessment using the PEDro scale

According to Moseley & Pinheiro (2022), the PEDro scale was developed in 1999 to rate studies that are indexed in the PEDro database (pedro.org.au). As of December 2021, ratings were available for a total of 40,256 studies. The scale comprises 11 items, each of which is assessed as present or absent. Ten of the items are used to calculate a summary score, known as the overall PEDro score (range 0 to 10), with higher scores indicating a lower risk of bias. One item (inclusion criterion and source) is not included in the overall score as it relates to external validity or generalisability and not risk of bias.

3.7.3 Evaluation using the CONSORT 2010 checklist

"The Consolidated Standards of Reporting Trials (CONSORT) Statement is a set of guidelines designed to improve the transparency and quality of reporting of randomised trials. It was first published in 1996, revised in 2001 and last updated in 2010 (Eldridge et al., 2016, cited in Schulz et al., 2010; Moher et al., 2010) and simultaneously published in 10 leading medical journals, including Lancet, JAMA, BMJ, Annals of Internal Medicine and PLoS Medicine. The CONSORT statement consists of a checklist of the minimum essential items that should be included in reports of randomised trials and a diagram documenting the progression of participants through the trial" (Eldridge et al., 2016). A checklist was created for each of the selected 10 RCTs, which is presented in tabular form. These tables (20-30) can be found from page 117 and in the appendix.

### 3.7.4 Assessment of the risk of bias (RoB1)

The Cochrane Risk of Bias (RoB1) tool was used to assess the biases in the included studies. According to Higgins et al. (2011), "errors in the design, conduct, analysis and reporting of randomised trials can lead to the effect of an intervention being underestimated or overestimated". The Cochrane Collaboration's risk of bias tool was developed to make this process more transparent and precise. The risk of bias tool comprises six categories of bias: Selection Bias, Performance Bias, Detection Bias, Attrition Bias, Reporting Bias and Other Bias. Within each category, assessments are made for one or more elements that may cover different aspects of the domain or different outcomes (Higgins et al., 2011).

### 3.7.5 Limitations

The limitations of the ten included RCTs were systematically analysed to ensure greater transparency. This analysis enables a precise assessment of the weaknesses of the studies and their potential influence on the results. The results of this analysis are described in detail and presented in tabular form in the results section of the paper. This structured presentation supports a clear overview and facilitates the comparison of the studies with regard to their methodological limitations.

CHAPTER 4

# 4 Overview of the studies

## 4.1 Population

Table 5 below shows the age of the test subjects (4.1.1), gender (4.1.2), recruitment strategy (4.1.3) and blinding (4.1.4):

Tab 5: Overview of the population of the included studies (own presentation 2024)

| Study | Age | Gender | Recruitment | Blinding |
|---|---|---|---|---|
| **Atan et al, 2020** | ST group: 44.67 ± 11.26 years; KT group: 49.80 ± 11.04 years | ST: 7 men, 8 women; KT: 6 men, 9 women | Clinic for Physical Medicine and Rehabilitation, Hitit University | Participants and outcome assessors blinded, clinicians not blinded |
| **Aydoga n et al., 2022** | 20-65 years | 28 women, 18 men | March 2020 until December 2021 | No blinding of practitioners, blinding of participants/outcome assessment not mentioned |
| **Delgado de la Sema et al, 2020** | 18-65 years | 25 men, 36 women | January to December 2017 | Outcome assessment blinded; patients may not be fully blinded |
| **Eladl et al, 2022** | 45-55 years | 65 % men, 35 % women | December 2018 until April 2019 | Patients and outcome assessment blinded, clinicians not blinded |
| **Fobbe et al, 2022** | 48.4 years (± 13 years) | 61.4 % Women | Clinic outpatient departments of theMHH (May 2020 to February 2021) | Physiotherapists blinded, investigators not blinded |
| **Michiel s et al, 2016** | 50 years (± 13 years) | Not specified | University Hospital Antwerp (tertiary tinnitus clinic) | Investigator and Therapists blinded |
| **Plaza-Monzan o et al, 2020** | 18-65 years | 25 men, 36 women | January to December 2017 | Outcome assessment blinded, subjects and practitioners not blinded |
| **T utar et al, 2020** | 41,17± 10.75 years | 22 men (36.7 %), 38 women (63.3 %) | January to December 2018, clinic in Turkey | Participants blinded, clinicians not blinded |
| **Van der Wal et al, 2020** | 45 years (± 14 years) | 53 % men, 47 % women | Antwerp University Hospital, Belgium | Practitioner blinded; Patients not blinded |
| **Zhe Yu et al, 2024** | 29.02 years (19-45 years) | 25 men (58.1 %), 18 women (41.9 %) | Eye and ENT Hospital, Fudan University (February to May 2019) | Assessor blinded; Subjects and practitioners not blinded |

## 4.2 Sample size

Table 6 below shows the number of subjects (4.2.1), the randomisation procedure (4.2.2), the exclusion of subjects and the reasons for exclusion (4.2.3) in the included studies.

Tab 6: Overview of the sample size of the included studies (own presentation 2024)

| Study | Number of test subjects | Randomisation method | Subject exclusion and reasons |
|---|---|---|---|
| **Atan et al, 2020** | 30 participants (ST: 15, KT: 15) | Random allocation with opaque envelopes | 7 participants cancelled; reasons: Lack of time, transport problems |
| **Aydogan et al, 2022** | 46 participants (TENS: 23, control group: 23) | Random allocation by computer programme | No reported exclusions |
| **Delgado de la Serna et al, 2020** | 61 participants (study group: 31, control group: 30) | Random allocation through computer-generated numbers | ENT pathologies, neurological diseases, previous CMD treatment |
| **Eladl et al, 2022** | 40 participants (study group: 20, control group: 20) | Block randomisation | Neurological diseases, hearing loss, orthopaedic contraindications |
| **Fobbe et al, 2022** | 80 participants (intervention group: 37, control group: 33) | Random allocation through sealed envelopes | 10 participants cancelled; reasons: Pandemic-related concerns (SARS-CoV-2) |
| **Michiels et al, 2016** | 38 participants (immediate start group: 19, Delay group: 19) | Block randomisation with variable block lengths, concealed Randomisation list | Two participants declined to participate after randomisation |
| **Plaza-Monzano et al, 2020** | 61 participants (study group: 31, control group: 30) | Random allocation through computer-generated numbers | ENT pathologies, neurological diseases, previous CMD treatment |
| **T utar et al, 2020** | 60 participants (3 groups, each with 20 participants) | Computerised randomisation | No reported dropouts |
| **Van der Wal et al, 2020** | 80 participants (early start group: 40, late start group: 40) | 1:1 block randomisation with variable block lengths | 5 dropouts: Follow-up not completed (3 early group, 2 late group) |
| **Zhe Yu et al, 2024** | 43 participants (immediate start group: 20, late start group: 23) | Random assignment through computer-generated randomisation | 3 participants could not be contacted; no feedback |

## 4.3 Inclusion and exclusion criteria

Table 7 below shows the inclusion and exclusion criteria of the included studies.

Tab 7: Inclusion and exclusion criteria of the included studies (own presentation 2024)

| Study | Inclusion criteria | Exclusion criteria |
|---|---|---|
| **Atan et al, 2020** | Patients with somatosensory tinnitus, neck complaints | Pregnancy, Middle ear diseases, operations |
| **Aydogan et al, 2022** | Normal hearing test, subjective chronic tinnitus | Pacemaker, previous ear surgery, abnormal hearing |
| **Delgado de la Serna et al,** | CMD-associated tinnitus, age 18-65 years | ENT pathologies, neurological diseases, contraindications for physiotherapy |

| | | |
|---|---|---|
| **2020** | | |
| **Eladl et al, 2022** | Patients with CST, restricted cervical ROM | Neurological diseases, orthopaedic contraindications |
| **Fobbe et al, 2022** | Adults with tinnitus and cervical spine complaints | Objective tinnitus, previous operations, cognitive impairments |
| **Michiels et al, 2016** | Chronic subjective tinnitus (TFI: 25-90), neck pain | Dizziness, objective tinnitus, severe mental disorders |
| **Plaza- IM onzano et al, 2020** | CMD-associated tinnitus, age 18-65 years | ENT pathologies, neurological diseases, contraindications for physiotherapy |
| **Tutar et al, 2020** | Age 18-65 years, chronic subjective tinnitus | Pregnancy, pacemaker, mental illness |
| **Van der Wal et al, 2020** | Adults with TFI score between 25-90; tinnitus stable | Otological causes, severe depression/anxiety, tumours |
| **Zhe Yu et al, 2024** | Diagnosed somatosensory tinnitus | Previous physiotherapy, psychiatric/neurological disorders |

### 4.4 Interventions

Table 8 below shows the type of group allocation (4.4.1), the interventions in the experimental group (4.4.2) and the control group (4.4.3), the implementation of the interventions (4.4.4), changes and modifications (4.4.5) as well as their type and reasons (4.4.5.1 and 4.4.5.2):

Tab 8: Overview of the interventions of the included studies (own presentation 2024)

| Study | Type of group assignment | Interventions in the experimental group | Interventions in the control group | Implementation of the interventions | Type of changes | Reasons for the changes |
|---|---|---|---|---|---|---|
| **Atan et al, 2020** | Randomised assignment to ST or KT group | Kinesio taping on sterno-cleidomastoid us, trapezius and levator scapulae | Placebo taping in neutral position | Once a week for four weeks | No changes reported | Not to meet |
| **Aydo gan et al, 2022** | Random Allocation | TENS therapy (20 sessions) | Information about tinnitus | 5 sessions per week over 4 weeks | No changes reported | Not to meet d |
| **Delga do de la Sern a et al, 2020** | Random Allocation | Movement, education and cervico-mandibular manual therapy | Movement and education | Six sessions within one month | None Change reported | Not to meet |
| **Eladl et al, 2022** | Random Allocation | PBMT + physiotherapeutic exercise programme | PBMT alone | Three sessions per week over eight weeks | No changes reported | Not to meet |
| **Fobb e et al., 2022** | Intervention group and control group | Manual therapy (thgger point therapy, stretching | Waiting list | An average of 17 sessions by certified therapists | No changes reported | Not to meet |

| | | | | | | |
|---|---|---|---|---|---|---|
| | | exercises) | | | | |
| **Michiels et al., 2016** | Immediate start group and delayed start group Pθ | Multimodal cervical physiotherapy | Delayed start: No treatment in the first 6 weeks | 12 sessions over 6 weeks | No changes reported | Not to meet |
| **Plaza -** | Random Allocation | Movement, education and | Movement and education | Six Meetings | No change | Notz u- |
| **Monzano et al., 2020** | | cervico-mandibular manual Therapy | | within of a month | reported | meet d |
| **Tutar et al, 2020** | Randomised into three groups | TENS on one or both ears | Placebo (no electrical or acoustic stimulation) | 10 sessions within one month | No changes reported | Not to meet |
| **Van der Wal et al, 2020** | Early start group vs. Late start group | Orofacial physiotherapy (including Muscle massage, exercises) | Delayed treatment after 9 weeks | Up to 18 sessions over a period of 9 weeks | No changes reported | Not to meet |
| **Zhe Yu et al, 2024** | Random Allocation | Physiotherapy Muscle training, stretching, mobilisation | No specific treatment | Individual therapy sessions of 60 minutes each, daily for 7 days | No changes reported | Not to meet |

## 4.5 Result measurement procedure

Table 9 below shows the primary outcome measures (4.5.1), the secondary outcome measures (4.5.2) and the measurement instruments used, including tests and questionnaires (4.5.3):

Tab 9: Outcome measurement methods of the included studies (own presentation 2024)

| **Study** | **Primary outcome measures** | **Secondary outcome measures** | **Measuring instruments (tests, questionnaires)** |
|---|---|---|---|
| **Atan et al, 2020** | Tinnitus Severity (VAS) | Tinnitus Handicap Inventory (THI), neck pain VAS, Neck Disability Index (NDI) | VAS, THI, NDI |
| **Aydogan et al, 2022** | Tinnitus Severity | VAS loudness and annoyance, THI (subscales: functional, emotional, catastrophic), SF-36 | VAS, THI, SF-36 |
| **Delgado de la Serna et al, 2020** | CMD pain (NPRS), tinnitus severity (VAS) | THI, CF-PDI, SF-12, BDI- II, PPT, range of motion of the mandible | NPRS, VAS, THI, CF-PDI, SF-12, BDI-II, pressure algometer |
| **Eladl et al, 2022** | Tinnitus intensity (VAS) | THI, cervical ROM (flexion, extension, lateral flexion, rotation) | VAS, THI, ROM measuring device |
| **Fobbe et** | Change in the Tinnitus | Change in muscle tone | THI, DHI, pressure pain |

| | | | |
|---|---|---|---|
| **al, 2022** | Handicap Inventory (THI), Dizziness Handicap Inventory (DHI) | | measurement, CROM device (mobility measurement of the cervical spine) |
| **Michiels et al, 2016** | Change in the Tinnitus Functional Index (TFI) | Change in the Neck Bournemouth Questionnaire (NBQ) and Global Perceived Effect (GPE) | TFI, NBQ, GPE |
| **Plaza-Monzano et al, 2020** | Tinnitus Severity (VAS), tinnitus handicap (THI) | Pressure pain thresholds (PPT), quality of life (SF-12), depression scores (BDI-II), range of motion of the mandible | VAS, THI, PPT, SF-12, BDI-II, plastic ruler |
| **T utar et al, 2020** | Change in the Tinnitus Handicap Index (THI) | Change in depression, anxiety and stress (DASS) | Turkish version of the THI, Depression Anxiety Stress Scales (DASS) |
| **Van der Wal et al, 2020** | Tinnitus Questionnaire (TQ) | Tinnitus Functional Index (TFI) | TQ, TFI |
| **Zhe Yu et al, 2024** | VAS (pain), THI (tinnitus impairment), NPRS (pain rating) | HCFA (history and characteristic functional activity) | THI, VAS, NPRS, HCFA |

CHAPTER 5

# 5 Results

## 5.1 Results of the PEDro scale

Table 10 below provides an overview of the included studies on the PEDro scale

Tab 10: The PEDro criteria of the included studies (own presentation 2024)

| | First author | 1 | 2 | 3 | 4 | 5 | 6 | 7 | 8 | 9 | 10 | 11 | Total |
|---|---|---|---|---|---|---|---|---|---|---|---|---|---|
| 1 | Atan 2020 | X | X | X | X | X | - | X | X | X | X | X | 9 |
| 2 | Aydogan 2022 | X | X | X | X | - | - | - | X | X | X | X | 7 |
| 3 | Delgado 2020 | X | X | X | X | - | - | X | X | X | X | X | 8 |
| 4 | Eladl 2022 | X | X | X | X | X | - | X | X | X | X | X | 9 |
| 5 | Fobbe 2022 | X | X | X | X | - | X | - | X | X | X | X | 8 |
| 6 | Michiels 2016 | X | X | X | X | - | X | X | X | X | X | X | 9 |
| 7 | Plaza-Manzano 2020 | X | X | X | X | - | - | - | X | X | X | X | 7 |
| 8 | Tutar 2020 | X | X | X | X | X | - | X | X | X | X | X | 9 |
| 9 | Van der Whale 2020 | X | X | X | X | - | X | - | X | X | X | X | 8 |
| 10 | Zhi Yu 2024 | x | x | x | x | - | - | x | x | x | x | x | 8 |

**PEDro criteria: 1**. the inclusion and exclusion criteria were specified **2**. randomised allocation of subjects **3.** concealed allocation of groups **4.** at the beginning of the study, the groups were similar with regard to the most important prognostic indicators **5.** blinding: subjects **6.** blinding: therapists **7.** blinding: investigators **8.** at least one key outcome was measured in more than 85% of the subjects originally allocated to the groups **9.** all subjects for whom the groups had been randomised were blinded to the outcome

Outcome measures were available, the treatment or control application was received as assigned or, if not, data for at least one key outcome were analysed by an intention to treat method **10.** Statistical group comparisons were reported for at least one key outcome **11.** The study reports both point and variability measures for at least one key outcome

## 5.2 CONSORT 2010 checklist

The completed CONSORT 2010 checklists of the ten included studies can be found in the appendix starting on page 117.

## 5.3 Results of the risk of bias assessment

5.3.1 Risk of bias: general overview (figure)

Fig 3 below shows an overview of the possible "risk of bias" of the included studies, based on the Cochrane Risk of Bias Tool (RoB1):

52Ta11

52Ta11

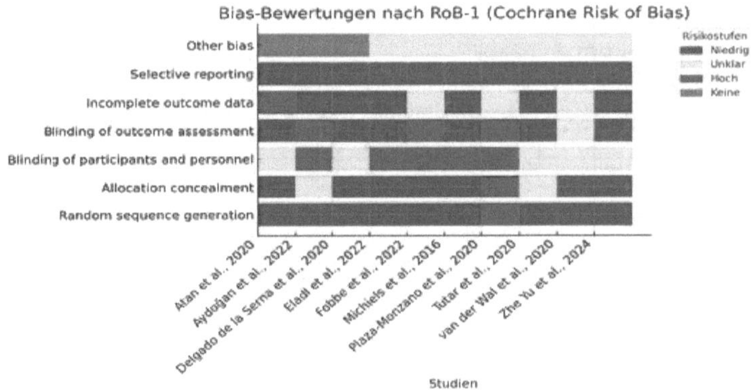


Fig 3: Risk of bias overview according to Cochrane RoB1 (own illustration 2024)

### 5.3.2 Risk of bias: overview of the individual studies

The following Table 11 shows an overview of possible "risk of bias" of the included studies based on the Cochrane Risk of Bias Tool (RoB1):

Tab 11: Risk of bias of the included studies (own presentation 2024)

| **Study** | **Category** | **Risk** | **Reason** |
|---|---|---|---|
| **Atan et al, 2020** | Random sequence generation (selection bias) | Low | Randomisation by computer and secrecy through sealed envelopes. |
| | Allocation concealment (selection bias) | Low | Sealed envelopes guarantee the confidentiality of the allocation. |
| | Blinding of participants and personnel (performance bias) | Moderate | The participants were blinded, but the treating physicians were not blinded. |
| | Blinding of outcome assessment (detection bias) | Low | Blinding of the outcome assessors ensured. |
| | Incomplete outcome data (attrition bias) | Moderate | 7 participants dropped out, reasons were given. |
| | Selective reporting (reporting bias) | Low | All planned endpoints were reported. |
| | Other bias | None | No further systematic biases identified. |
| **Study** | Category | Risk | Reason |
| **Aydogan et al, 2022** | Random sequence generation (selection bias) | Low | Randomised allocation ensured by computer program. |
| | Allocation concealment (selection bias) | Moderate | Details on the confidentiality of the assignment were not clearly stated. |
| | Blinding of participants and personnel (performance bias) | High | Treaters were not allied. |
| | Blinding of outcome assessment (detection bias) | High | Blinding of the outcome assessment not mentioned. |

| | | | |
|---|---|---|---|
| | Incomplete outcome data (attrition bias) | Low | No reported failures. |
| | Selective reporting (reporting bias) | Low | Results were reported completely and transparently. |
| | Other bias | None | No other sources of bias identified. |
| **Study** | Category | Risk | Reason |
| **Delgado de la Serna et al, 2020** | Random sequence generation (selection bias) | Low | Randomised allocation with concealed envelopes ensured. |
| | Allocation concealment (selection bias) | Low | Concealed allocation guaranteed. |
| | Blinding of participants and personnel (performance bias) | Moderate | Patients may not have been completely blinded; investigators were not blinded. |
| | Blinding of outcome assessment (detection bias) | Low | Outcome assessment carried out by blinded experts. |
| | Incomplete outcome data (attrition bias) | Low | No failures reported. |
| | Selective reporting (reporting bias) | Low | Results were reported completely and transparently. |
| | Other bias | None | No further systematic biases identified. |
| **Author** | Bias category | Risk | Reason |
| **Eladl et al, 2022** | Random sequence generation (selection bias) | Low | Random allocation was performed by computer-generated block randomisation with concealed allocation. |
| | Allocation concealment (selection bias) | Low | Concealed allocation guaranteed. |
| | Blinding of participants and personnel (performance bias) | High | The treatment providers were not allied, which allows for possible differences in the intervention. |
| | Blinding of outcome assessment (detection bias) | Low | The measurement of earnings was allied, which minimised the risk of measurement distortions. |
| | Incomplete outcome data (attrition bias) | Low | All participants were analysed until the end of the study; no failures were reported. |
| | Selective reporting (reporting bias) | Low | All defined endpoints were reported completely and transparently. |
| | Other bias | Medium | No long-term follow-up period; potential gender-specific differences were not analysed. |
| **Author** | Bias category | Risk | Reason |
| **Fobbe et al, 2022** | Random sequence generation (selection bias) | Low | Randomised allocation ensured by opaque envelopes. |
| | Allocation concealment (selection bias) | Low | Group assignment concealed and randomly organised by envelopes. |
| | Blinding of participants | High | Participants were not blinded, which |

| | | | |
|---|---|---|---|
| | and personnel (performance bias) | | could potentially influence the results. |
| | Blinding of outcome assessment (detection bias) | High | Investigator was not blinded, which increases the risk of subjective evaluation. |
| | Incomplete outcome data (attrition bias) | Moderate | Dropouts explained by pandemic, but potential influence on study results not ruled out. |
| | Selective reporting (reporting bias) | Low | Complete reporting of the results. |
| | Other bias | Medium | No complete blinding and possibility of a placebo effect. |
| **Author** | Bias category | Risk | Reason |
| **Michiels et al, 2016** | Random sequence generation (selection bias) | Low | Randomised assignment with hidden randomisation list. |
| | Allocation concealment (selection bias) | Low | Hidden group assignment guaranteed by encrypted randomisation list. |
| | Blinding of participants and personnel (performance bias) | High | Participants knew about group membership. |
| | Blinding of outcome assessment (detection bias) | Low | Alliance of the therapists and the examiner ensured. |
| | Incomplete outcome data (attrition bias) | Low | Two dropouts, but well documented. |
| | Selective reporting (reporting bias) | Low | Complete reporting of all results. |
| | Other bias | Medium | Possibility of a placebo effect due to the lack of a control group without active treatment. |
| **Author** | Bias category | Risk | Reason |
| **Plaza-Monzano et al, 2020** | Random sequence generation (selection bias) | High | Lack of information on randomisation and concealed allocation. |
| | Allocation concealment (selection bias) | High | Lack of transparent presentation of allocation procedures. |
| | Blinding of participants and personnel (performance bias) | High | No alliance of the practitioners. |
| | Blinding of outcome assessment (detection bias) | High | No alliance of the investigators. |
| | Incomplete outcome data (attrition bias) | Moderate | Dropout rates and reasons were not fully reported. |
| | Selective reporting (reporting bias) | Low | All predefined endpoints were reported. |
| | Other bias | Moderate | Possible bias due to insufficient sample size and lack of blinding of |

| | | | |
|---|---|---|---|
| | | | randomisation. |
| **Author** | Bias category | Risk | Reason |
| **Tutar et al, 2020** | Random sequence generation (selection bias) | Low | Randomisation is carried out using a computer-generated programme. |
| | Allocation concealment (selection bias) | Moderate | No sufficient documentation on blinding of group allocation available. |
| | Blinding of participants and personnel (performance bias) | Moderate | No blinding of the practitioners. |
| | Blinding of outcome assessment (detection bias) | Low | Participants were allied and results were measured consistently. |
| | Incomplete outcome data (attrition bias) | Low | No dropouts reported. |
| | Selective reporting (reporting bias) | Low | All predefined endpoints were reported. |
| | Other bias | Moderate | Methodological limitations and potential influence of placebo effects cannot be ruled out. |
| **Author** | Bias category | Risk | Reason |
| **van der Wal et al, 2020** | Random sequence generation (selection bias) | Low | Block randomisation with variable block lengths and hidden randomisation list by an independent evaluator. |
| | Allocation concealment (selection bias) | Low | Concealed allocation with an independent assessor ensured. |
| | Blinding of participants and personnel (performance bias) | Moderate | Treaters were allied, but nothing mentioned about blinding of participants. |
| | Blinding of outcome assessment (detection bias) | Moderate | It is unclear whether the results were assessed by blinded examiners. |
| | Incomplete outcome data (attrition bias) | Moderate | Dropout rate of 5 participants, but documented with clear justification. |
| | Selective reporting (reporting bias) | Low | All pre-specified endpoints were reported. |
| | Other bias | Moderate | Possible bias due to lack of comparison group for placebo effects and recruitment from tertiary care. |
| **Author** | Bias category | Risk | Reason |
| **Zhe Yu et al, 2024** | Random sequence generation (selection bias) | Low | Randomised allocation of participants using a computer-generated programme. |
| | Allocation concealment (selection bias) | Low | Allocation concealment ensured by concealed allocation. |
| | Blinding of participants and personnel (performance bias) | Moderate | No double blinding, subjects were not blinded, but therapists were blinded. |
| | Blinding of outcome | Low | Results were analysed by blinded raters. |

| | | | |
|---|---|---|---|
| | assessment (detection bias) | | |
| | Incomplete outcome data (attrition bias) | Low | Dropout rate below 10 %, detailed information available on the reasons for the exclusion of participants. |
| | Selective reporting (reporting bias) | Low | All pre-registered endpoints were reported in the study. |
| | Other bias | Moderate | Possible bias due to small sample size and short follow-up period. |

## 5.4 Limitations of the included RCTs

Table 12 below shows the limitations of the included studies:

Tab 12: Limitations of the included studies (own presentation 2024)

| Study | Limitation | details |
|---|---|---|
| **Atan et al, 2020** | Small sample size | Only 30 patients, which limits generalisability. |
| | Short follow-up period | Only 4 weeks follow-up. |
| | Specific patient selection | Only patients with somatosensory tinnitus and neck complaints were included. |
| | No long-term effects investigated | Long-term effects of the intervention not assessed. |
| **Aydogan et al, 2022** | No alliance of practitioners | Introduction of performance bias possible. |
| | Allocation of the results assessment unclear | Potential bias in the collection of results. |
| | Short follow-up period | Long-term effects of TENS therapy not investigated. |
| | Heterogeneous Participant charact erist ics | Different Initial conditions could influence results. |
| **Delgado de La Serna et al, 2020** | No control group without intervention | Natural course of the disease not taken into account. |
| | Potential placebo effect not investigated | No sham therapy group available. |
| | No objective Diagnostic method for tinnitus | Diagnoses are based exclusively on self-reports. |
| | Patient expectations | Possible influence of expectations regarding manual therapy on the results. |
| **Eladl et al, 2022** | Short follow-up period | Only 8 weeks follow-up time, no long-term results available. |
| | Lack of alliance | Investigators were not allied, potential bias. |
| | Restricted population | Only patients aged 45 to 55 years, limited generalisability. |
| | Subjective measuring instruments | Primary results are based on self-reporting (VAS, THI). |
| | Individual treatment centres | Data from one centre (Cairo University), reduced transferability. |

| | | |
|---|---|---|
| | No placebo control | Control group received no placebo intervention. |
| **Fobbe et al, 2022** | Missing placebo control group | No comparison with placebo or alternative therapy. |
| | Partial lack of alliance | Participants and investigators not allied, potential bias. |
| | Variability of techniques | Different manual techniques by therapists. |
| | Dropouts due to the pandemic | SARS-CoV-2 infection fears, potential impact on outcomes. |
| | Subjective endpoints | Results are based on self-reporting by participants (THI, DHI). |
| **Michiels et al, 2016** | No placebo control group | No comparison with control group without intervention. |
| | Limited sample size | Only 38 participants, results to be confirmed. |
| | Short follow-up period | Effectiveness over longer periods unclear. |
| | Not complete<br>Allying the participants | Participants knew about<br>Group membership. |
| | Variability in treatment | Therapists were able to customise techniques, heterogeneity in intervention. |
| **Plaza- Monzano et al, 2020** | Lack of an alliance | Participants, therapists and investigators were not blinded. |
| | Potential selection bias | No details on the concealed allocation of participants. |
| | Generability | Results not transferable to other populations. |
| | Limited long-term data | No follow-up data or long-term results reported. |
| | Small sample size | Only 61 participants, limited informative value. |
| **Tutar et al, 2020** | No long-term data | Long-term effect of TENS not investigated. |
| | Lack of a<br>Double blinding | Participants were blinded, but not the practitioner. |
| | Limited generalisability | Results may not be transferable. |
| | Small sample size | Only 60 participants, limited informative value. |
| **Van der Wal et al, 2020** | Delayed treatment design | Comparison of the groups only possible in week 9, underestimated effect of the treatment. |
| | No comparative treatment | Placebo effects not excluded. |
| | Recruitment from tertiary care | Results may not be transferable to primary care. |
| | Lack of double blinding | Potential performance bias due to lack of blinding of subjects and practitioners. |
| | No stratification according to | Results could be influenced by |

| | | |
|---|---|---|
| | tinnitus severity | differences in tinnitus severity at baseline. |
| **Zhe Yu et al, 2024** | Small sample size | Only 43 participants, reduced generalisability. |
| | Follow-up data | No follow-up data for late start group. |
| | No placebo control group | Placebo effects cannot be ruled out. |
| | Lack of<br>Long-term observation | Long-term effects beyond 12 weeks have not been investigated. |
| | Blinding | Potential bias due to lack of blinding of the test subjects. |

## 5.5 Study results

5.5.1 Overview of the study results

Tables 13 to 19 below show the primary and secondary outcomes of all ten RCTs relevant to the Master's thesis.

Tab 13: Tinnitus severity (VAS), (own illustration 2024)

| Authors | Group | Baseline value (mean ± SD) | Final value (mean ± SD) | Difference (final value - initial value) | p- value |
|---|---|---|---|---|---|
| **Atan et al.** | KT Group | 7,47 ± 1,24 | 5,07 ± 1,33 | -2,40 | <0,001 |
| | ST Group | 7,13 ± 2,26 | 6,58 ± 1,88 | -0,55 | 0,108 |

| | | | | | |
|---|---|---|---|---|---|
| **Aydogan et al.** | TENS group | 6,34 ± 1,89 | 3,34 ± 2,36 | -3,00 | 0,001 |
| | Control group | 6,04 ± 2,09 | 6,00 ± 1,40 | -0,04 | 0,800 |
| **Delgado et al.** | Movement+ Education | 6,70 ± 1,20 | 5,80 ± 1,20 | -0,90 | <0,001 |
| | Movement + education + manual therapy | 6,80 ± 1,20 | 4,70 ± 1,90 | -2,10 | <0,001 |
| **Eladl et al.** | Group A | 7,44 ± 0,69 | 3,60 ± 0,82 | -3,84 | 0,001 |
| | Group B | 7,25 ±0,71 | 5,65 ± 1,13 | -1,60 | 0,001 |
| **Plaza-Monzano et al.** | Movement + Training | 6,80 ± 1,50 | 5,20 ± 1,30 | -1,60 | 0,002 |
| | Exercise + training + manual therapy | 6,70 ± 1,40 | 3,10 ± 1,20 | -3,60 | 0,002 |
| **T utar et al.** | Group A | 6,80 ± 1,50 | 5,15 ± 1,30 | -1,65 | 0,001 |
| | Group B | 6,90 ± 1,40 | 4,35 ± 1,20 | -2,55 | 0,001 |
| | Group C | 6,70 ± 1,60 | 6,45 ± 1,70 | -0,25 | 0,05 |
| **van der Wal et al.** | Early start group | 50 ±30 | 46 ±28 | -4 | 0,042 |
| | Late start group | 49 ±25 | 48 ±26 | -1 | 0,721 |
| **Zhe Yu et al.** | Instant start group | 3,95 ± 1,93 | 2,40 ± 1,00 | -1,55 | 0,005 |
| | Late start group | 4,22 ± 1,95 | 3,95 ± 1,90 | -0,27 | 0,342 |

| **Authors** | **Group** | **Baseline value (mean ± SD)** | **Final value (mean ± SD)** | **Difference (final value - initial value t)** | **p-value** |
|---|---|---|---|---|---|
| **Atan et al.** | KT Group | 65,73 ± 10,84 | 52,67 ± 13,02 | -13,06 | 0,001 |
| | ST Group | 61,06 ± 17,72 | 59,33 ± 17,80 | -1,73 | 0,500 |
| **Aydoga n et al.** | TENS group | 38,78 ±23,50 | 22,69 ± 18,83 | -16,09 | 0,001 |
| | Control group | 50,15 ± 13,45 | 48,35 ± 23,79 | -1,80 | 0,600 |
| **Delgado et al.** | Movement+ Education | 34,20 ± 11,90 | 28,30 ± 11,80 | -5,90 | <0,001 |
| | Movement + education + Manual therapy | 36,10 ±9,50 | 14,40 ± 7,30 | -21,70 | <0,001 |
| **Eladl et al.** | Group A | 46,30 ± 7,61 | 31,05 ± 4,43 | -15,25 | 0,001 |
| | Group B | 45,90 ± 8,23 | 36,40 ± 5,40 | -9,50 | 0,001 |
| **Fobbe et al.** | Intervention group | 43,00 ± 19,00 | 22,30 ± 21,72 | -20,70 | <0,001 |
| | Control group | 45,60 ±21,72 | 41,60± 21,72 | -4,00 | 0,423 |

| | | | | | |
|---|---|---|---|---|---|
| **Michiels et al.** | Instant start group | 50,00 ± 23,00 | 33,10 ± 20,00 | -16,90 | 0,001 |
| | Delay start group | 51,00 ± 18,00 | 49,00 ± 18,00 | -2,00 | 0,055 |
| **Plaza-Monzan o et al.** | Exercise + training | 45,30 ± 12,10 | 37,40 ± 10,60 | -7,90 | <0,00 1 |
| | Exercise + training + manual therapy | 46,00 ± 12,80 | 30,20 ± 12,00 | -15,80 | <0,00 1 |
| **T utar et al.** | Group A | 37,80 ± 20,70 | 10,20 ± 8,90 | -27,60 | 0,001 |
| | Group B | 35,10±21,10 | 8,60 ± 4,90 | -26,50 | 0,001 |
| | Group C | 37,90 ± 21,00 | 28,70 ± 15,00 | -9,30 | 0,001 |

Tab 15: Numerical pain rating scale (NRPS), (own illustration 2024)

| **Autore n** | **Group** | **Baseline value (mean ± SD)** | **Final value (mean ± SD)** | **Difference (final value - initial value)** | **p-value** |
|---|---|---|---|---|---|
| **Delgad o et al.** | Movement + education | 5,20 ± 1,70 | 3,60 ± 1,50 | -1,60 | <0,00 1 |
| | Movement + education + Manual therapy | 5,20 ± 2,20 | 2,20 ± 1,50 | -3,00 | <0,00 1 |
| **Zhe Yu et al.** | Instant start group | 3,84 ± 2,00 | 2,55 ± 0,89 | -1,29 | 0,025 |
| | Delay start group | 4,13 ± 2,07 | 3,50 ± 1,91 | -0,63 | 0,308 |

Tab 16: Neck Bournemouth Questionnaire (NBQ), (own illustration 2024)

| **Autore n** | **Group** | **Baseline value (mean ± SD)** | **Final value (mean ± SD)** | **Difference (final value - initial value)** | **p-value** |
|---|---|---|---|---|---|
| **Michiel s et al.** | Instant start group | 37,00 ± 10,00 | 18,68 ± 12,00 | -18,32 | <0,00 1 |
| | Delay start group | 32,00 ± 12,00 | 25,62 ± 15,00 | -6,38 | 0,041 |

Tab 17: Neck Disability Index (NDI), (own presentation 2024)

| **Authors** | **Group** | **Baseline value (mean ± SD)** | **Final value (mean ± SD)** | **Difference (final value - initial value)** | **p- value** |
|---|---|---|---|---|---|
| **Atan et al.** | KT Group | 19,53 ±6,62 | 12,80 ±5,08 | -6,73 | 0,001 |
| | ST Group | 23,47 ± 5,33 | 23,47 ± 5,46 | 0,00 | 0,500 |
| **Delgado et al.** | Movement+ Education | 19,00 ±5,00 | 15,00 ±4,00 | -4,00 | 0,002 |
| | Movement+ Education + Manual therapy | 18,00 ± 6,00 | 10,00 ± 3,00 | -8,00 | <0,001 |

Tab 18: Tinnitus function index (TFI), (own presentation 2024)

| Autore n | Group | Baseline (mean ± SD) | Final value (mean ± SD) | Difference (final value - initial value ) | p-value |
|---|---|---|---|---|---|
| **Michiel s et al.** | Instant start group | 50,00 ± 23,00 | 33,10 ± 20,00 | -16,90 | 0,001 |
| | Delay start group | 51,00 ± 18,00 | 49,00 ± 18,00 | -2,00 | 0,055 |
| **van der Wal et al.** | Early start group | 55,00 ± 17,00 | 39,00 ± 14,00 | -16,00 | 0,042 |
| | Late start group | 48,00 ± 15,00 | 36,00 ± 13,00 | -12,00 | 0,721 |

Tab 19: Tinnitus questionnaire (TQ), (own illustration 2024)

| Authors | Group | Baseline value (mean ± SD) | Final value (mean ± SD) | Difference (final value - initial value) | p-value |
|---|---|---|---|---|---|
| **van der Wal et al.** | Early start group | 37,00 ± 16,00 | 31,00± 14,00 | -6,00 | 0,042 |
| | Late start group | 34,00 ± 15,00 | 30,00 ± 14,00 | -4,00 | 0,099 |

5.5.2 Results of the individual studies

For the sake of clarity and transparency, the results of the ten selected RCTs, including the demographic characteristics of the participants and all primary and secondary outcomes, are presented in detail in the appendix. The relevant information can be found in Tables 30 to 62 from page 142 onwards.

CHAPTER 6

# 6 Discussion

## 6.1 Discussion of the results

The primary research question of this thesis addresses the effectiveness of physiotherapy interventions in the treatment of tinnitus associated with CMD or upper cervical spine. To answer this question, ten RCTs were selected that investigated different therapeutic approaches in randomised groups to evaluate the effectiveness of physiotherapy interventions.

The measures analysed include

Physiotherapeutic exercises/exercise programmes, movement

Manual therapy, cervicomandibular manual therapy

TENS (transcutaneous electrical nerve stimulation)

PBMT (photobiomodulation therapy)

Kinesio taping, sham taping

Placebo interventions

Orofacial physiotherapy

Multimodal cervical physiotherapy

Muscle training

Trigger point therapy and stretches

Education/Education

The results show that physiotherapy interventions, especially in combination with other treatment modalities, can bring about significant improvements in patients with CMD- or cervical spine-associated tinnitus.

The RCT by **Delgado et al. (2020)** examined 61 patients with CMD-associated tinnitus who were randomised into two groups:

□ KT group (control group): Physiotherapy consisting of exercises and information/education.

□ ST group: Physiotherapy as in the KT group, supplemented by cervico-mandibular manual therapy.

Both groups received six sessions over a period of one month. After a follow-up of six months, the results showed clear differences:

The tinnitus severity (VAS) fell from 6.8 to 2.8 points in the ST group, while only a reduction to 4.7 points was achieved in the KT group.

The THI score was significantly reduced by 21.7 points in the ST group, compared to only 5.9 points in the KT group.

These results make it clear that additional manual therapy significantly increases the effectiveness of the multimodal approach and represents an important supplement to standard physiotherapy.

The RCT by **Eladl et al. (2022)** examined a total of 52 patients with CST who were randomised into two groups:

PBMT group: 26 patients who only received PBMT.

PBMT+physiotherapy group: 26 patients who received PBMT combined with a supervised physiotherapy exercise programme.

The results showed that the PBMT+physiotherapy group achieved significantly greater improvements:

THI score: reduction of 20.5 points compared to 12.3 points in the PBMT group.

□ VAS pain intensity: Decrease of 3.7 points compared to 2.1 points in the PBMT group.

□ Neck range of motion (ROM): Increase of 15° compared to 8° in the PBMT group.

These results show that the combination of PBMT and physiotherapy is more effective for

CST than PBMT alone and that multimodal approaches should be favoured.

The RCT by **Fobbe et al. (2022)** examined 54 patients with CST and vertigo symptoms who were randomised into two groups:

□ Intervention group (IG): 27 patients received manual therapy.

□ Control group (CG): 27 patients without specific intervention.

Results:

□ THI values: IG: reduction from 40.7 to 22.3 ($\Delta = 18$, $p < 0.001$, $r = 0.47$); KG: only slight changes.

□ DHI values: IG: reduction from 34.00 to 12.77 ($\Delta = 21.23$, $p = 0.010$, $r = 0.49$); KG: no significant changes.

□ Hypertonus of the right splenius capitis muscle: IG: decrease from 34 to 12 patients ($p < 0.001$, Phi = 0.562); KG: no changes.

These results show the effectiveness of manual therapy for CST and vertigo symptoms. Fobbe et al. emphasise the need for future studies to further investigate long-term effects and the role of specific muscles.

The RCT by **Michiels et al. (2016)** examined 38 patients with cervicogenic somatic tinnitus (CST) who were randomised into two groups:

□ Immediate start therapy group: 19 patients immediately received multimodal cervical physiotherapy (12 sessions over 6 weeks).

□ Retard therapy group: 19 patients received the same therapy after a 6-week waiting period.

Results:

□ TFI responses to treatment: All patients ($n = 38$) suffered from severe tinnitus at the start of the study with an average TFI score of 49 points (SD: 21). Immediately after treatment, the TFI score dropped significantly to 44 points ($p = 0.04$), but rose again to 47 points after 6 weeks of follow-up.

□ NBQ scores: The average NBQ score decreased from 33 points (baseline) to 16 points after treatment ($p < 0.001$) and increased slightly to 21 points after follow-up, but remained significantly improved ($p = 0.001$).

□ Perceived global effect (GPE): After 6 weeks of baseline measurement, 58% of patients in the immediate start group (11 out of 19) reported a significant improvement in tinnitus, compared to no improvement in the delayed treatment group. Immediately after treatment, 53% of the total study population (20 out of 38) experienced a significant improvement in tinnitus. After 6 weeks of follow-up, this effect persisted in 24% of patients (9 out of 38).

Conclusion: The results show that multimodal cervical physiotherapy can bring about significant short-term improvements in all patients with severe tinnitus. After the follow-up period, this effect persisted in just under a quarter of patients. Given the chronicity and treatment resistance of the symptoms in the tertiary referral centre population studied, these success rates can be considered remarkable. However, long-term effects require further research.

Similar to the RCT by Michiels et al. (2016), **Côté et al. (2019)** came to the conclusion in their study with a quasi-experimental pre-post design that a multimodal physiotherapy programme can achieve significant improvements in patients with somatosensory tinnitus. The 6-week programme included cervical and thoracic mobilisations, muscle strengthening, stretching, postural instruction and stabilisation. The programme involved 31 adults who received an average of 10 treatments.

Results:

□ THI reduction: -15 points ($p < 0.001$ )

□ VAS-L (tinnitus loudness): -13 points ($p < 0.001$)

□ VAS-A (tinnitus annoyance): -15 points ($p < 0.001$)
□ VAS-C (neck pain): -21 points ($p < 0.001$)
□ NDI (cervical functional impairment): -9 points ($p < 0.001$)

Of the 31 participants, 14 people (45%) showed a significant improvement in their tinnitus, which was also maintained after 3 months. Positive indicators for the success of the therapy were the absence of a family history of tinnitus, recent onset of tinnitus and somatosensory modulations.

Conclusion: The results confirm the effectiveness of multimodal physiotherapy approaches in patients with somatosensory tinnitus and complement the findings of Michiels et al. (2016). Future studies with larger samples could help to further validate the long-term effectiveness and prognostic indicators.

The RCT by **van der Wal et al. (2020)** investigated the effect of multidisciplinary orofacial treatment on patients with temporomandibular somatosensory tinnitus. Patients were randomised into an early start group (n = 40) and a delayed start group (n = 40). The treatment comprised orofacial physiotherapy with a focus on muscle relaxation, postural adjustment, jaw exercises and, if necessary, occlusal splints.

Results:

□ Tinnitus Functional Index (TFI): Early start group: reduction of 13.8 points after treatment ($p = 0.042$). Delayed start group: reduction of 12.2 points after treatment.

Follow-up: Clinically relevant improvement in 61% of patients.

□ Tinnitus Questionnaire (TQ): Early start group: 30% of patients showed a decrease in TQ score of at least one grade, compared to 2.8% in the delayed start group ($p = 0.006$).

□ Long-term effect: Both groups showed an additional improvement in the follow-up period, which indicates that the treatment had a lasting effect.

Conclusion: The results show that multidisciplinary, non-invasive orofacial treatment can significantly reduce the severity of TST. This study supports the effectiveness of physiotherapeutic approaches for temporomandibular tinnitus and emphasises the importance of multimodal therapies.

The RCT by **Zhe Yu et al. (2024)** investigated the effectiveness of physiotherapy in patients with somatosensory tinnitus, especially in severe cases. A total of 80 patients** were randomised into an immediate start group (n = 40) and a control group (n = 40). The intervention consisted of physiotherapy treatments focussing on the head and neck region.

Results:

□ VAS values (tinnitus loudness): Baseline (both groups): 6.5 ± 1.2 points.After 1 week of treatment: immediate start group: reduction to 3.8 ± 1.1 points ($\Delta = -2.7$, $p < 0.01$ ). Control group: No significant change (6.4 ± 1.3 points).

□ Tinnitus Handicap Inventory (THI): Baseline score (both groups): 50 ± 12 points. After 1 week of treatment: Immediate start group: reduction to 34 ± 10 points ($\Delta = -16$, $p < 0.01$). Control group: No significant change (49 ± 13 points).

□ Numerical Pain Rating Scale (NPRS): baseline score (both groups): 5.8 ± 1.0 points. After 1 week of treatment: immediate start group: reduction to 2.5 ± 0.9 points ($\Delta = -3.3$, $p < 0.01$). Control group: No significant change (5.7 ± 1.1 points).

□ Long-term effects (after 12 weeks): 35 % of patients in the immediate start group continued to show stable improvements in all measured parameters (VAS, THI, NPRS).

Conclusion: The results show that targeted physiotherapeutic treatment of the head and neck region leads to significant and lasting improvements in patients with somatosensory tinnitus.

**Aydogan et al. (2022)** and **Tutar et al. (2020)** conducted randomised controlled trials to investigate the efficacy of transcutaneous electrical nerve stimulation (TENS) for somatosensory tinnitus.

□ Study design and participants:

**Aydogan et al (2022):** Participants: 46 (TENS group: n = 23, control group: n = 23). Intervention: TENS (20 sessions over 4 weeks) versus education only in the control group.

**Tutar et al (2020):** Participants: 60, randomised into three groups: Unilateral TENS stimulation: n = 20, Bilateral TENS stimulation: n = 20 and placebo: n = 20. Intervention: 10 sessions over 1 month.

Results:

THI:

**Aydogan et al:** TENS group: 38.78 ± 23.50 to 22.69 ± 18.83 (Δ = -16.09, p = 0.001). Control group: no significant change.

**Tutar et al.:** Significantly lower THI values in the TENS groups compared to the placebo group (p < 0.05).

VAS (tinnitus loudness):

**Aydogan et al.:** 6.34 ± 1.89 to 3.34 ± 2.36 (Δ = -3.0, p = 0.001 ).

Quality of life:

**Aydogan et al:** Improved subjective quality of life in the TENS group.

DASS (Depression-Anxiety-Stress-Scale):

**Tutar et al.:** Significant improvements in the TENS groups compared to the placebo group (p < 0.05).

Conclusion: Both studies confirm that TENS is an effective, safe and practicable method to: Reduce THI and VAS and improve quality of life and psychological well-being (DASS). These results emphasise the benefits of TENS as a promising treatment option for chronic subjective tinnitus.

A prospective study by **Buergers et al. (2014)** investigated the relationship between CMD and tinnitus and the effectiveness of physiotherapy and occlusal splints in patients with CMD and tinnitus.

The study carried out the interventions in 2 groups: CMD group (n = 91, 36.6% with tinnitus) and control group without CMD (n = 91, 4.4% with tinnitus) comparing the effects of physiotherapy and occlusal splints on CMD-associated tinnitus.

Results: Tinnitus prevalence: CMD: 36.6 % vs. Control group: 4.4 % (p < 0.001)

□ Tinnitus localisation: With unilateral CMD, tinnitus always occurred on the same side.

□ Treatment results:

Physiotherapy: improvement or complete remission in 50% of patients.

Bite splint: improvement or complete remission in 33% of patients

Conclusions: The results show that physiotherapy is more effective than occlusal splints for CMD-associated tinnitus and is a promising treatment option.

A placebo-controlled study by **Campagna et al. (2021)** investigated the effectiveness of dry needling (DN) in patients with chronic somatosensory tinnitus and myofascial trigger points (MTP). The placebo group consisted of 8 participants, as did the intervention group (DN group).

DN group: n = 8, four weekly sessions in which myofascial trigger points were specifically treated with DN.

Placebo group: n = 8, placebo DN without actual stimulation of the trigger points.

Results:

□ THI reduction: DN group: -10.75 points (p = 0.024)

□ Emotional stress: significant improvement (p = 0.011)

□ Placebo group: No significant changes

Conclusion: Dry needling showed significant improvements in tinnitus handicap and emotional distress. However, due to the small sample size, the significance remains limited, which is why further large-scale studies are required.

### 6.2 Conclusion of the discussion

The results of the 10 RCTs analysed confirm the hypothesis posed in the primary research question that physiotherapy is effective for tinnitus associated with CMD and upper cervical spine disorders. In these studies, various physiotherapeutic measures were carried out in randomised groups and analysed as comparative or additional therapy.

Several studies of different designs are available in the literature, most of which included at least one form of physiotherapy and achieved positive results. The results of the studies by Côté, Campagna and Buergers are consistent with the RCTs analysed and also demonstrate the significant effectiveness of physiotherapy. This emphasises the importance of this form of treatment as a central component of multimodal approaches that focus not only on reducing the burden of tinnitus, but also on improving functional and psychological parameters.

### 6.3 Limitations of the study situation

The literature search in the Medline (PubMed & PMC), PEDro and ScienceDirect databases was continued throughout the entire period of the Master's thesis until shortly before its completion. The aim was to identify the most recently published studies that address the specific questions of this thesis and include at least the components of physiotherapy, tinnitus and CMD or cervical spine. However, it was noticeable that only a small number of RCTs exist that specifically addressed tinnitus in conjunction with CMD or the upper cervical spine. Even rarer were RCTs that also investigated physiotherapy interventions as a treatment option. This limitation made the selection of suitable literature considerably more difficult and stretched the planned time frame of the search.

Similarly, Fabrizia et al. (2024) reported comparable limitations in the study situation in their systematic review and meta-analysis. The authors investigated the effectiveness of different treatment approaches for tinnitus associated with CMD based on only five RCTs with a total of 329 participants that were suitable for meta-analysis - a strikingly small number. The meta-analysis showed that a multidisciplinary, non-invasive approach is most effective, especially for patients with moderate to severe tinnitus, and described physiotherapy as the most effective treatment of choice for somatic tinnitus and CMD-related symptoms. At the same time, methodological weaknesses such as small samples, short follow-up periods and a high degree of heterogeneity in the treatment methods were identified in the analysis, which also point to the need for further high-quality studies.

Finally, due to this limited study situation, only a manageable number of ten RCTs could be identified that are closest to the topic of the research question and provide insights into the effectiveness of physiotherapy for somatosensory tinnitus. In order to obtain more evidence and generalisable results, future large-scale RCTs are needed that include both longer follow-up periods and larger samples, as well as a wider range of interventions. These should systematically compare physiotherapy interventions with other approaches such as splints, drug therapy, shockwave therapy, injections, acupuncture, laser, placebo and other available interventions in randomised two- or multi-arm groups. Multimodal physiotherapy approaches should also be investigated more intensively in order to better understand their combined effectiveness.

CHAPTER 7

# 7 Conclusion

This master's thesis emphasises the central importance of physiotherapy as an effective treatment option for CMD, cervical spine disorders and the associated somatosensory tinnitus. The results of the analysed studies not only show therapeutic success, but also highlight the urgency of further strengthening evidence-based research in this area.

Tinnitus is not only a considerable burden for those affected, but also a relevant factor for the health economy. According to Tziridis et al. (2022), annual healthcare costs in Germany average EUR 2206.95 per patient. With a prevalence of 5.5% and around 4.57 million people affected, the total annual costs add up to between EUR 21.9 and 35.4 billion. Comparable studies from the USA, the UK and the Netherlands confirm similar annual costs per patient. These figures show that tinnitus is not only an individual burden, but also an economic challenge - comparable to diseases such as COPD (16 billion euros) or diabetes mellitus (52 billion euros per year).

Fabrizia et al (2024) confirm in their systematic review and meta-analysis that CMD and cervical spine problems are among the most common causes of somatosensory tinnitus. They emphasise that physiotherapy is often the most effective treatment option, both by providing significant symptom relief and by identifying predictive factors that can improve treatment outcomes.

The research question of this thesis is highly relevant for physiotherapy as it addresses common and widespread complaints such as CMD, cervical spine dysfunctions and tinnitus. These problems are related to increasing environmental and psychosocial stress, the intensive use of multimedia devices and the prevalence of sedentary behaviour. The hypothesis that physiotherapy is an effective treatment option for somatosensory tinnitus has been clearly confirmed by the results of high-quality studies with robust data.

In conclusion, it can be stated that there are still significant gaps in the current study situation, particularly in the area of randomised controlled trials. This opens up new opportunities for physiotherapy to expand its evidence base through methodologically high-quality studies with larger samples and innovative approaches. The integration of different interventions could not only further demonstrate the effectiveness of physiotherapy, but also strengthen its role as a key player in the treatment and prevention of CMD, cervical spine and tinnitus-related complaints. In this way, physiotherapy can consolidate its importance on a practical and scientific level in the long term and help to significantly improve the quality of life of those affected.

## BIBLIOGRAPHY

Ahmad SA, Hasan S, Saeed S, Khan A, Khan M. Low-level laser therapy for temporomandibular joint disorders: a systematic review. J Med Live. 2021 MarchApril; 14(2):148-164. DOI: 10.25122/JML-2020-0169. PMID: 34104237; PMCID: PMC8169142.

Atan, Tugba; Atan, Dogan; Özel, Sumru (2020): Effectiveness of Kinesio taping in the treatment of somatosensory tinnitus: A randomised controlled trial. In: Complementary therapies in clinical practice 39, p. 101100. DOI: 10.1016/j.ctcp.2020.101100.

Aydogan, Zehra; Satekin, Merve Cinar; Uyar, Muhammed Sefa; Aksoy, Songül; Tokgoz-Yilmaz, Suna (2022): Transcutaneous Electric Nerve Stimulation in Chronic Subjective Tinnitus. In: American journal of otolaryngology 43 (5), p. 103521. DOI: 10.1016/j.amjoto.2022.103521.

Biesinger, E.; Groth, A.; Höing, R.; Hölzl, M. (2015): Somatosensory tinnitus. In: Hno 63 (4), pp. 266-271. DOI: 10.1007/s00106-014-2971-9.

Böhni, U. W. (2014): Diagnosis of dysfunction and therapy of the upper cervical region. In: Manual Medicine 52 (3), pp. 251-268. DOI: 10.1007/s00337-014-1108-2.

Bordoni B, Varacallo M. Anatomy, head and neck, temporomandibular joint. 2023 July 17. In: StatPearls [Internet]. Treasure Island (FL): StatPearls Publishers; 2024 Jan-. PMID: 30860721.

Bousema, E. J.; Koops, E. A.; van Dijk, P.; Dijkstra, P. U. (2018): Association Between Subjective Tinnitus and Cervical Spine or Temporomandibular Disorders: A Systematic Review. In: Trends in Hearing 22. DOI: 10.1177/2331216518800640.

Bousema, Eric J.; Koops, Elouise A.; van Dijk, Pim; Dijkstra, Pieter U. (2023): Effects of Physical Interventions on Subjective Tinnitus, a Systematic Review and Meta-Analysis. In: Brain Sciences 13 (2). DOI: 10.3390/brainsci13020226.

Buergers R, Kleinjung T, Behr M, Vielsmeier V. Is there a connection between tinnitus and temporomandibular joint disorders? J Protheset Dent. 2014 Mar; 111(3):222-7. doi: 10.1016/j.prosdent.2013.10.001. Epub 25 November 2013. PMID: 24286640. Dalrymple Sarah N.; Lewis, Sarah H.; Philman, Samantha (2021): Tinnitus: Diagnosis and Management. In: American family physician 103 (11), pp. 663-671.

Campagna CA, Anauate J, Vasconrelos LGE, Oiticica J. Efficacy of dry needling for bothersome chronic tinnitus in patients with myofascial trigger points. Int Arch Otorhinolaryngol. 30 August 2021; 26(2): e233-e242. DOI: 10.1055/S-0041- 1730429. PMID: 35602278; PMCID: PMC9122774.

Côté C, Baril I, Morency CÈ, Montminy S, Couture M, Leblond J, Roos M, Roy JS. Long-term effects of a multimodal physiotherapy programme on the severity of somatosensory tinnitus and identification of clinical indicators predicting favourable programme outcomes. J Am Acad Audiol. 2019 September; 30(8):720-730. DOI: 10.3766/jaaa.17147. PMID: 31526469.

Da Silva, Marianne Trajano; Silva, Carlos; Silva, Jade; Costa, Mateus; Gadotti, Inae; Ribeiro, Karyna (2023): Effectiveness of Physical Therapy Interventions for Temporomandibular Disorders Associated with Tinnitus: A Systematic Review. In: Journal of Clinical Medicine 12 (13). DOI: 10.3390/jcm12134329.

de Oliveira LRLB, Alves IDS, Vieira APF, Passos UL, Leite CDC, Gebrim ES. Temporomandibular joint: from anatomy to internal derangement. Radiol BHs. 2023 March-April; 56(2):102-109. DOI: 10.1590/0100-3984.2022.0072-en. PMID: 37168044; PMCID: PMC10165975.

Delgado de La Serna, Pablo; Plaza-Manzano, Gustavo; Cleland, Joshua; Fernández- de-Las-Peñas, César; Martín-Casas, Patricia; Díaz-Arribas, María José (2020): Effects of Cervico-Mandibular Manual Therapy in Patients with Temporomandibular Pain Disorders and Associated Somatic Tinnitus: A Randomised Clinical Trial. In: Pain medicine (Malden, Mass.)

21 (3), pp. 613-624. DOI: 10.1093/pm/pnz278.
Eladl, Hadaya Mosaad; Elkholi, Safaa M.; Eid, Marwa M.; Abdelbasset, Walid Kamal; Ali, Zeinab A.; Bahey El-Deen, Heba A. (2022): Effect of adding a supervised physical therapy exercise program to photobiomodulation therapy in the treatment of cervicogenic somatosensory tinnitus: A randomised controlled study. In: Medicine 101 (31). DOI: 10.1097/MD.0000000000029946.
Fabrizia, d' Apuzzo; Giuseppe, Minervini; Martina, Cerbone; Patricia, Rotolo Rossana; Vincenzo, Grassia; Ludovica, Nucci (2024): Treatment approaches, outcomes and prognostic indicators in patients with tinnitus and temporomandibular disorders evaluated with DC/TMD: A systematic review and Meta-analysis. In: Journal of oral rehabilitation. DOI: 10.1111/joor.13796.
Fobbe, A.; Bökel, A.; Lesinski-Schiedat, A.; Gutenbrunner, C.; Sturm, C. (2022): Pilot study: manual medical method evaluation on the modulability of the leading symptom tinnitus: a prospective randomised study. In: *Hno 70 (9), p.* 675684. DOI: 10.1007/s00106-022-01198-2.
Gçbska, Magdalena; Dalewski, Bartosz; Palka, Lukasz; Kotodziej, Lukasz (2023): Evaluation of the efficacy of manual soft tissue therapy and therapeutic exercises in patients with pain and limited mobility TMJ: a randomised control trial (RCT). In: Head & Face Medicine 19. DOI: 10.1186/s13005-023-00385-y.
Gil-Martínez, Alfonso; Paris-Alemany, Alba; López-de-Uralde-Villanueva, Ibai; La Touche, Roy (2018): Management of pain in patients with temporomandibular disorder (TMD): challenges and solutions. In: Journal of Pain Research 11, pp. 571-587. DOI: 10.2147/JPR.S127950.
Haider, Haúla F.; Hoare, Derek J.; Costa, Raquel F. P.; Potgieter, Iskra; Kikidis, Dimitris; Lapira, Alec et al. (2017): Pathophysiology, Diagnosis and Treatment of Somatosensory Tinnitus: A Scoping Review. In: Frontiers in neuroscience 11, p. 207. DOI: 10.3389/fnins.2017.00207.
Higgins, Julian P. T.; Altman, Douglas G.; G0tzsche, Peter C.; Jüni, Peter; Moher, David; Oxman, Andrew D. et al. (2011): The Cochrane Collaboration's tool for assessing risk of bias in randomised trials. In: BMJ 343, d5928. DOI: 10.1136/bmj.d5928.
Koparal, Mehtap; Sirik, Mehmet; Yavuz, Gunay Yapici; Ege, Bilal (2022): Evaluation of the relationship between temporomandibular joint disorders and tinnitus with computed tomography. In: Journal of stomatology, oral and maxillofacial surgery 123 (4), e199- e205. DOI: 10.1016/j.jormas.2022.06.015.
La Hernández-Nuño de Rosa, María F.; Keith, David A.; Siegel, Noah S.; Moreno-Hay, Isabel (2022): Is there an association between otologic symptoms and temporomandibular disorders? An evidence-based review. In: Journal of the American Dental Association (1939) 153 (11), pp. 1096-1103. DOI: 10.1016/j.adaj.2021.07.029.
Langguth, Berthold; Elgoyhen, Ana Belen; Cederroth, Christopher R. (2019): Therapeutic Approaches to the Treatment of Tinnitus. In: Annual review of pharmacology and toxicology 59, pp. 291-313. DOI: 10.1146/annurev-pharmtox-010818- 021556.
Langguth, Berthold; Ridder, Dirk de; Schlee, Winfried; Kleinjung, Tobias (2024): Tinnitus: Clinical Insights into Its Pathophysiology-A Perspective. In: Journal of the Association for Research in Otolaryngology: JARO 25 (3), pp. 249-258. DOI: 10.1007/s10162-024-00939-0.
Lina-Granade, G.; Truy, E.; Ionescu, E.; Garnier, P.; Thai Van, H. (2016): Acouphènes et articulation temporo-mandibulaire : état des connaissances. In: Revue de stomatologie, de chirurgie maxillo-faciale et de chirurgie orale 117 (6), pp. 458-462. DOI: 10.1016/j.revsto.2016.10.005.
Li, Dion Tik Shun; Leung, Yiu Yan (2021): Temporomandibular Disorders: Current Concepts and Controversies in Diagnosis and Management. In: Diagnostics 11 (3). DOI:

10.3390/diagnostics11030459.
Lomas, Jonathan; Gurgenci, Taylan; Jackson, Christopher; Campbell, Duncan (2018): Temporomandibular dysfunction. In: Australian journal of general practice 47 (4), pp. 212-215. DOI: 10.31128/AFP-10-17-4375.
Ma, Xiaoyan; Wang, Fangyuan; Zhang, Chi; Shen, Weidong; Yang, Shiming (2022): Self-Directed Neurofeedback Treatment for Subjective Tinnitus Patients Evaluated by Multimodal Functional Imaging. In: Neural Plasticity 2022. DOI: 10.1155/2022/5114721.
Meulemeester, Kayleigh de; Meeus, Mira; Pauw, Robby de; Cagnie, Barbara; Keppler, Hannah; Lenoir, Dorine (2023): Suffering from chronic tinnitus, chronic neck pain, or both: Does it impact the presence of signs and symptoms of central sensitisation? In: PloS one 18 (8). DOI: 10.1371/journal.pone.0290116.
Michiels, S.; van de Heyning, P.; Truijen, S.; Hallemans, A.; Hertogh, W. de (2016): Does multi-modal cervical physical therapy improve tinnitus in patients with cervicogenic somatic tinnitus? In: Manual therapy 26, pp. 125-131. DOI: 10.1016/j.math.2016.08.005.
Michiels, S.; van de Heyning, P.; Truijen, S.; Hallemans, A.; Hertogh, W. de (2017): Prognostic indicators for decrease in tinnitus severity after cervical physical therapy in patients with cervicogenic somatic tinnitus. In: Musculoskeletal science & practice 29, pp. 33-37. DOI: 10.1016/j.msksp.2017.02.008.
Michiels, Sarah (2023): Somatosensory Tinnitus: Recent Developments in Diagnosis and Treatment. In: Journal of the Association for Research in Otolaryngology: JARO 24 (5), pp. 465-472. DOI: 10.1007/s10162-023-00912-3.
Michiels, Sarah; Ganz Sanchez, Tanit; Oron, Yahav; Gilles, Annick; Haider, Haúla F.; Erlandsson, Soly et al. (2018): Diagnostic Criteria for Somatosensory Tinnitus: A Delphi Process and Face-to-Face Meeting to Establish Consensus. In: Trends in Hearing 22. DOI: 10.1177/2331216518796403.
Miyamoto-Aldave, Toshi-Hiromi; Asmat-Abanto, Angel-Steven; Ulloa-Cueva, Delia-Margarita; Minchón-Medina, Carlos-Alberto; Llanos-Vera, Víctor-Eduardo; Callirgos- Briones, Jannette-Vanessa (2024): Temporomandibular joint dysfunction in relation to tinnitus in Peruvian patients: A cross-sectional study. In: Journal of Clinical and Experimental Dentistry 16 (4), e448-54. DOI: 10.4317/jced.61358.
Moseley, Anne M.; Pinheiro, Marina B. (2022): Research Note: Evaluating risk of bias in randomised controlled trials. In: *Journal of physiotherapy* 68 (2), pp. 148-150. DOI: 10.1016/j.jphys.2022.02.003.
Oostendorp, Rob A. B.; Bakker, Iem; Elvers, Hans; Mikolajewska, Emilia; Michiels, Sarah; Hertogh, Willem de; Samwel, Han (2016): Cervicogenic somatosensory tinnitus: An indication for manual therapy? Part 2: Clinical evaluation. In: Manual therapy 23, pp. 124-127. DOI: 10.1016/j.math.2015.11.009.
Patil, Jayaditya Devpal; Alrashid, Manar Abdulkarim; Eltabbakh, Ayah; Fredericks, Salim (2023): The association between stress, emotional states, and tinnitus: a mini-review. In: Frontiers in Aging Neuroscience 15. DOI: 10.3389/fnagi.2023.1131979.
Pelicioli, Marcelo; Myra, Rafaela Simon; Florianovicz, Vivian Carla; Batista, Juliana Secchi (2017): Physiotherapeutic treatment in temporomandibular disorders. In: Revista Dor 18 (4). DOI: 10.5935/1806-0013.20170129.
Plaza-Manzano, Gustavo; Delgado-de-la-Serna, Pablo; Díaz-Arribas, María J.; Rodrigues-de-Souza, Diana P.; Fernández-de-Las-Peñas, César; Alburquerque- Sendín, Francisco (2021): Influence of Clinical, Physical, Psychological, and Psychophysical Variables on Treatment Outcomes in Somatic Tinnitus Associated with Temporomandibular Pain: Evidence From a Randomized Clinical Trial. In: *Pain practice the official journal of World Institute of Pain* 21 (1), pp. 8-17. DOI: 10.1111/papr.12919.
Ralli, Massimo; Greco, Antonio; Boccassini, Armando; Altissimi, Giancarlo; Di Paolo, Carlo;

Falasca, Vincenzo et al. (2018): Subtyping patients with somatic tinnitus: Modulation of tinnitus and history for somatic dysfunction help identify tinnitus patients with temporomandibular joint disorders. In: PloS one 13 (8). DOI: 10.1371/journal.pone.0202050.

Rethlefsen, Melissa L.; Page, Matthew J. (2022): PRISMA 2020 and PRISMA-S: common questions on tracking records and the flow diagram. In: Journal of the Medical *Library Association: JMLA* 110 (2), pp. 253-257. DOI: 10.5195/jmla.2022.1449.

Tsang, Benjamin K. T.; Collins, Grant G.; Anderson, Shane; Westcott, Myriam (2024): Tinnitus update: what can be done for the ringing? In: Internal medicine journal 54 (7), pp. 1066-1076. DOI: 10.1111/imj.16414.

Tutar, Belgin; Atar, Sevgi; Berkiten, Güler; Üstün, Onur; Kumral, Tolgar Lütfi; Uyar, Yavuz (2020): The effect of transcutaneous electrical nerve stimulation (TENS) on chronic subjective tinnitus. In: *American journal of otolaryngology* 41 (1), p. 102326. DOI: 10.1016/j.amjoto.2019.102326.

Tziridis, Konstantin; Friedrich, Jana; Brüeggemann, Petra; Mazurek, Birgit; Schulze, Holger (2022): Estimation of Tinnitus-Related Socioeconomic Costs in Germany. In: *Int. J. Env. Res. Pub. He.* 19 (16). DOI: 10.3390/ijerph191610455.

Urbariski P, Trybulec B, Pihut M. The use of manual techniques in masticatory muscle relaxation as an adjunct therapy in the treatment of temporomandibular joint disorders. Int J Environ Res Public Health. 8 December 2021; 18(24):12970. DOI: 10.3390/ijerph182412970. PMID: 34948580; PMCID: PMC8700844.

van der Wal, Annemarie; Michiels, Sarah; van de Heyning, Paul; Braem, Marc; Visscher, Corine; Topsakal, Vedat et al. (2020): Treatment of Somatosensory Tinnitus: A Randomized Controlled Trial Studying the Effect of Orofacial Treatment as Part of a Multidisciplinary Program. In: *Journal of clinical medicine* 9 (3). DOI: 10.3390/JCM9030705.

Wadhwa, Smriti; Jain, Shraddha; Patil, Nimisha; Jungade, Shyam (2024): Cervicogenic Somatic Tinnitus: A Narrative Review Exploring Non-otologic Causes. In: Cureus 16 (7), e65476. DOI: 10.7759/cureus.65476.

Wagner, Florian Max-Josef (2022): Somatic dysfunction of the cervical spine and its complex clinical picture: principles of manual medical diagnosis of cervicobrachialgia and cervicocephalic syndrome. In: Der Orthopäde 51 (4), p. 263273. DOI: 10.1007/s00132-022-04228-7.

Xiong, Xin; Gao, Xinlin; Zhong, Jiawei; Hu, Shoushan; Li, Yijun; Zheng, Yunhao; Liu, Yang (2023): Bibliometric Analysis of Research on Temporomandibular Joint and Occlusion from 2000 to 2022. In: Journal of Pain Research 16, pp. 2847-2860. DOI: 10.2147/JPR.S418362.

1. search protocol of the literature search in Medline (PubMed and PMC)

Zhe Yu, Gong JM, Hong GW, Zhou RQ, Fu XP, Fan T, Zheng YQ, Peng YQ, Li J, Wang YF. The effect of physiotherapy on somatosensory tinnitus. J Clin Med. 14 June 2024; 13(12):3496. DOI: 10.3390/JCM13123496. PMID: 38930025; PMCID: PMC11204550.

ANNEX

1. Fig 4 below shows the search protocol for the literature search in Medline (PubMed and PMC)

# History and Search Details

download

Delete

| Search | Actions | details | Query | Results | Time |
|---|---|---|---|---|---|
| #35 | | | Search: (((((((therapeutic exercise) OR (physical rehabilitation)) OR (manual therapy)) OR (manual therapy)) OR (physical therapy)) OR (physiotherapy)) AND (((((((((neck related tinnitus) OR (cervicogenic tinnitus)) OR (cervical tinnitus)) OR (somatic tinnitus)) OR (somatosensory tinnitus)) OR (subjective tinnitus)) OR (ear noise)) OR (ear ringing)) OR (tinnitus))) AND (((((((((((((temporomandibular disorder) OR (tmd)) OR (temporomandibular dysfunction)) OR (cmd)) OR (craniomandibular dysfunction)) OR ((craniomandibular disorder) AND (temporomandibular joint dysfunction))) OR (temporomandibular joint syndrome)) OR (jaw disorders)) OR (cervicocephalic region)) OR (cervical spine)) OR (upper cervical vertebrae)) OR (upper cervical spine))) Filters: Full text, Randomised Controlled Trial, from 2012-2024 | 7 | 13:32:26 |
| #44 | | | Search: (((((((therapeutic exercise) OR (physical rehabilitation)) OR (manual therapy)) OR (manual therapy)) OR (physical therapy)) OR (physiotherapy)) AND (((((((((neck related tinnitus) OR (cervicogenic tinnitus)) OR (cervical tinnitus)) OR (somatic tinnitus)) OR (somatosensory tinnitus)) OR (subjective tinnitus)) OR (ear noise)) OR (ear ringing)) OR (tinnitus))) AND (((((((((((((temporomandibular disorder) OR (tmd)) OR (temporomandibular dysfunction)) OR (cmd)) OR | 7 | 13:32:09 |
| | | | (craniomandibular dysfunction)) OR ((craniomandibular disorder) AND (temporomandibular joint dysfunction))) OR (temporomandibular joint syndrome)) OR (jaw disorders)) OR | | |

| | | | | | |
|---|---|---|---|---|---|
| | | | (cervicocephalic region)) OR (cervical spine)) OR (upper cervical vertebrae)) OR (upper cervical spine))) Filters: Full text, Randomised Controlled Trial, from 2010-2024 | | |
| #43 | | | Search: (((((((therapeutic exercise) OR (physical rehabilitation)) OR (manual therapy)) OR (manual therapy)) OR (physical therapy)) OR (physiotherapy)) AND (((((((((neck related tinnitus) OR (cervicogenic tinnitus)) OR (cervical tinnitus)) OR (somatic tinnitus)) OR (somatosensory tinnitus)) OR (subjective tinnitus)) OR (ear noise)) OR (ear ringing)) OR (tinnitus))) AND (((((((((((((temporomandibular disorder) OR (tmd)) OR (temporomandibular dysfunction)) OR (cmd)) OR (craniomandibular dysfunction)) OR ((craniomandibular disorder) AND (temporomandibular joint dysfunction))) OR (temporomandibular joint syndrome)) OR (jaw disorders)) OR (cervicocephalic region)) OR (cervical spine)) OR (upper cervical vertebrae)) OR (upper cervical spine))) Filters: Full text, from 2010 - 2024 | 59 | 13:31:49 |
| #42 | | | Search: (((((((therapeutic exercise) OR (physical rehabilitation)) OR (manual therapy)) OR (manual therapy)) OR (physical therapy)) OR (physiotherapy)) AND (((((((((neck related tinnitus) OR (cervicogenic tinnitus)) OR (cervical tinnitus)) OR (somatic tinnitus)) OR (somatosensory tinnitus)) OR (subjective tinnitus)) OR (ear noise)) OR (ear ringing)) OR (tinnitus))) AND (((((((((((((temporomandibular disorder) OR (tmd)) OR (temporomandibular dysfunction)) OR (cmd)) OR (craniomandibular dysfunction)) OR ((craniomandibular disorder) AND (temporomandibular joint dysfunction))) OR (temporomandibular joint syndrome)) OR (jaw disorders)) OR (cervicocephalic region)) OR (cervical | 62 | 13:31:20 |
| | | | spine)) OR (upper cervical vertebrae)) OR (upper cervical spine))) Filters: from 2010 - 2024 | | |

| | | | | | |
|---|---|---|---|---|---|
| #31 | | | Search: (((((((therapeutic exercise) OR (physical rehabilitation)) OR (manual therapy)) OR (manual therapy)) OR (physical therapy)) OR (physiotherapy)) AND (((((((((neck related tinnitus) OR (cervicogenic tinnitus)) OR (cervical tinnitus)) OR (somatic tinnitus)) OR (somatosensory tinnitus)) OR (subjective tinnitus)) OR (ear noise)) OR (ear ringing)) OR (tinnitus))) AND ((((((((((((temporomandibular disorder) OR (tmd)) OR (temporomandibular dysfunction)) OR (cmd)) OR (craniomandibular dysfunction)) OR ((craniomandibular disorder) AND (temporomandibular joint dysfunction))) OR (temporomandibular joint syndrome)) OR (jaw disorders)) OR (cervicocephalic region)) OR (cervical spine)) OR (upper cervical vertebrae)) OR (upper cervical spine))) | 101 | 13:28:33 |
| #41 | | | Search: (((((((therapeutic exercise) OR (physical rehabilitation)) OR (manual therapy)) OR (manual therapy)) OR (physical therapy)) OR (physiotherapy)) AND (((((((((neck related tinnitus) OR (cervicogenic tinnitus)) OR (cervical tinnitus)) OR (somatic tinnitus)) OR (somatosensory tinnitus)) OR (subjective tinnitus)) OR (ear noise)) OR (ear ringing)) OR (tinnitus))) AND ((((((((((((temporomandibular disorder) OR (tmd)) OR (temporomandibular dysfunction)) OR (cmd)) OR (craniomandibular dysfunction)) OR ((craniomandibular disorder) AND (temporomandibular joint dysfunction))) OR (temporomandibular joint syndrome)) OR (jaw disorders)) OR (cervicocephalic region)) OR (cervical spine)) OR (upper cervical vertebrae)) OR (upper cervical spine))) Filters: Randomised Controlled Trial | 9 | 13:28:26 |
| #37 | | | Search: (((((((therapeutic exercise) OR (physical rehabilitation)) OR (manual therapy)) OR (manual therapy)) OR (physical therapy)) OR | 8 | 13:28:21 |
| | | | (physiotherapy)) AND (((((((((neck | | |

| | | | | | |
|---|---|---|---|---|---|
| | | | related tinnitus) OR (cervicogenic tinnitus)) OR (cervical tinnitus)) OR (somatic tinnitus)) OR (somatosensory tinnitus)) OR (subjective tinnitus)) OR (ear noise)) OR (ear ringing)) OR (tinnitus))) AND ((((((((((((temporomandibular disorder) OR (tmd)) OR (temporomandibular dysfunction)) OR (cmd)) OR (craniomandibular dysfunction)) OR ((craniomandibular disorder) AND (temporomandibular joint dysfunction))) OR (temporomandibular joint syndrome)) OR (jaw disorders)) OR (cervicocephalic region)) OR (cervical spine)) OR (upper cervical vertebrae)) OR (upper cervical spine))) Filters: Full text, Randomised Controlled Trial | | |
| #36 | | | Search: (((((((therapeutic exercise) OR (physical rehabilitation)) OR (manual therapy)) OR (manual therapy)) OR (physical therapy)) OR (physiotherapy)) AND (((((((((neck related tinnitus) OR (cervicogenic tinnitus)) OR (cervical tinnitus)) OR (somatic tinnitus)) OR (somatosensory tinnitus)) OR (subjective tinnitus)) OR (ear noise)) OR (ear ringing)) OR (tinnitus))) AND ((((((((((((temporomandibular disorder) OR (tmd)) OR (temporomandibular dysfunction)) OR (cmd)) OR (craniomandibular dysfunction)) OR ((craniomandibular disorder) AND (temporomandibular joint dysfunction))) OR (temporomandibular joint syndrome)) OR (jaw disorders)) OR (cervicocephalic region)) OR (cervical spine)) OR (upper cervical vertebrae)) OR (upper cervical spine))) Filters: Free full text, Full text, Randomised Controlled Trial, from 2012-2024 | 2 | 13:27:59 |
| #40 | | | Search: (((((((therapeutic exercise) OR (physical rehabilitation)) OR (manual therapy)) OR (manual therapy)) OR (physical therapy)) OR (physiotherapy)) AND (((((((((neck related tinnitus) OR (cervicogenic tinnitus)) OR (cervical tinnitus)) OR (somatic tinnitus)) OR (somatosensory tinnitus)) OR | 9 | 13:26:45 |

| | | | | | |
|---|---|---|---|---|---|
| | | | (subjective tinnitus)) OR | | |
| | | | (ear noise)) OR (ear ringing)) OR (tinnitus))) AND ((((((((((((temporomandibular disorder) OR (tmd)) OR (temporomandibular dysfunction)) OR (cmd)) OR (craniomandibular dysfunction)) OR ((craniomandibular disorder) AND (temporomandibular joint dysfunction))) OR (temporomandibular joint syndrome)) OR (jaw disorders)) OR (cervicocephalic region)) OR (cervical spine)) OR (upper cervical vertebrae)) OR (upper cervical spine))) Filters: Free full text, Randomised Controlled Trial, Review | | |
| #39 | | | Search: (((((((therapeutic exercise) OR (physical rehabilitation)) OR (manual therapy)) OR (manual therapy)) OR (physical therapy)) OR (physiotherapy)) AND (((((((((neck related tinnitus) OR (cervicogenic tinnitus)) OR (cervical tinnitus)) OR (somatic tinnitus)) OR (somatosensory tinnitus)) OR (subjective tinnitus)) OR (ear noise)) OR (ear ringing)) OR (tinnitus))) AND ((((((((((((temporomandibular disorder) OR (tmd)) OR (temporomandibular dysfunction)) OR (cmd)) OR (craniomandibular dysfunction)) OR ((craniomandibular disorder) AND (temporomandibular joint dysfunction))) OR (temporomandibular joint syndrome)) OR (jaw disorders)) OR (cervicocephalic region)) OR (cervical spine)) OR (upper cervical vertebrae)) OR (upper cervical spine))) Filters: Free full text, Randomised Controlled Trial, from 2012-2024 | 2 | 13:26:35 |
| #38 | | | Search: (((((((therapeutic exercise) OR (physical rehabilitation)) OR (manualtherapy)) OR (manual therapy)) OR (physical therapy)) OR (physiotherapy)) AND (((((((((neck related tinnitus) OR (cervicogenic tinnitus)) OR (cervical tinnitus)) OR (somatic tinnitus)) OR (somatosensory tinnitus)) OR (subjective tinnitus)) OR (ear noise)) OR (ear ringing)) OR | 7 | 13:25:27 |

| | | | | | |
|---|---|---|---|---|---|
| | | | (tinnitus))) AND ((((((((((((temporomandibular disorder) OR (tmd)) OR (temporomandibular | | |
| | | | dysfunction)) OR (cmd)) OR (craniomandibular dysfunction)) OR ((craniomandibular disorder) AND (temporomandibular joint dysfunction))) OR (temporomandibular joint syndrome)) OR (jaw disorders)) OR (cervicocephalic region)) OR (cervical spine)) OR (upper cervical vertebrae)) OR (upper cervical spine))) Filters: Abstract, Full text, Randomised Controlled Trial, from 2012-2024 | | |
| #34 | | | Search: (((((((therapeutic exercise) OR (physical rehabilitation)) OR (manual therapy)) OR (manual therapy)) OR (physical therapy)) OR (physiotherapy)) AND (((((((((neck related tinnitus) OR (cervicogenic tinnitus)) OR (cervical tinnitus)) OR (somatic tinnitus)) OR (somatosensory tinnitus)) OR (subjective tinnitus)) OR (ear noise)) OR (ear ringing)) OR (tinnitus))) AND ((((((((((((temporomandibular disorder) OR (tmd)) OR (temporomandibular dysfunction)) OR (cmd)) OR (craniomandibular dysfunction)) OR ((craniomandibular disorder) AND (temporomandibular joint dysfunction))) OR (temporomandibular joint syndrome)) OR (jaw disorders)) OR (cervicocephalic region)) OR (cervical spine)) OR (upper cervical vertebrae)) OR (upper cervical spine))) Filters: Full text, from 2012 - 2024 | 57 | 12:43:58 |
| #33 | | | Search: (((((((therapeutic exercise) OR (physical rehabilitation)) OR (manual therapy)) OR (manual therapy)) OR (physical therapy)) OR (physiotherapy)) AND (((((((((neck related tinnitus) OR (cervicogenic tinnitus)) OR (cervical tinnitus)) OR (somatic tinnitus)) OR (somatosensory tinnitus)) OR (subjective tinnitus)) OR (ear noise)) OR (ear ringing)) OR (tinnitus))) AND ((((((((((((temporomandibular disorder) OR (tmd)) OR (temporomandibular dysfunction)) OR (cmd)) OR | 59 | 12:43:45 |

| | | | | | |
|---|---|---|---|---|---|
| | | | (craniomandibular dysfunction)) OR ((craniomandibular disorder) AND (temporomandibular joint dysfunction))) OR (temporomandibular joint | | |
| | | | syndrome)) OR (jaw disorders)) OR (cervicocephalic region)) OR (cervical spine)) OR (upper cervical vertebrae)) OR (upper cervical spine))) Filters: from 2012 - 2024 | | |
| #32 | | | Search: (((((((therapeutic exercise) OR (physical rehabilitation)) OR (manual therapy)) OR (manual therapy)) OR (physical therapy)) OR (physiotherapy)) AND (((((((((neck related tinnitus) OR (cervicogenic tinnitus)) OR (cervical tinnitus)) OR (somatic tinnitus)) OR (somatosensory tinnitus)) OR (subjective tinnitus)) OR (ear noise)) OR (ear ringing)) OR (tinnitus))) AND ((((((((((((temporomandibular disorder) OR (tmd)) OR (temporomandibular dysfunction)) OR (cmd)) OR (craniomandibular dysfunction)) OR ((craniomandibular disorder) AND (temporomandibular joint dysfunction))) OR (temporomandibular joint syndrome)) OR (jaw disorders)) OR (cervicocephalic region)) OR (cervical spine)) OR (upper cervical vertebrae)) OR (upper cervical spine))) Filters: from 2013 - 2024 | 59 | 12:43:34 |
| #30 | | | Search: (((((therapeutic exercise) OR (physical rehabilitation)) OR (manual therapy)) OR (manual therapy)) OR (physical therapy)) OR (physiotherapy) | 686,037 | 12:40:11 |
| #29 | | | Search: ((((((((neck related tinnitus) OR (cervicogenic tinnitus)) OR (cervical tinnitus)) OR (somatic tinnitus)) OR (somatosensory tinnitus)) OR (subjective tinnitus)) OR (ear noise)) OR (ear ringing)) OR (tinnitus) | 26,616 | 12:39:17 |
| #28 | | | Search: ((((((((((((temporomandibular disorder) OR (tmd)) OR (temporomandibular dysfunction)) OR (cmd)) OR (craniomandibular dysfunction)) OR ((craniomandibular disorder) AND (temporomandibular joint dysfunction))) OR (temporomandibular joint syndrome)) OR (jaw disorders)) | 123,902 | 12:37:55 |

| | | | | | |
|---|---|---|---|---|---|
| | | | OR (cervicocephalic region)) OR (cervical spine)) OR (upper cervical vertebrae)) OR (upper cervical spine)) | | |
| #27 | | | Search: therapeutic exercise | 176,906 | 12:35:40 |
| #26 | | | Search: physical rehabilitation | 286,816 | 12:35:09 |
| #25 | | | Search: manualtherapy | 15 | 12:34:34 |
| #24 | | | Search: manual therapy | 51,262 | 12:33:46 |
| #23 | | | Search: physical therapy | 436,393 | 12:33:32 |
| #22 | | | Search: physiotherapy | 250,509 | 12:33:17 |
| #21 | | | Search: cervicocephalic region | 55 | 12:32:56 |
| #20 | | | Search: cervical spine | 68,006 | 12:32:26 |
| #19 | | | Search: upper cervical vertebrae | 5,207 | 12:32:07 |
| #18 | | | Search: upper cervical spine | 7,684 | 12:31:40 |
| #17 | | | Search: neck related tinnitus | 897 | 12:31:05 |
| #16 | | | Search: cervicogenic tinnitus | 32 | 12:30:47 |
| #15 | | | Search: cervical tinnitus | 4,220 | 12:30:22 |
| #14 | | | Search: somatic tinnitus | 218 | 12:30:06 |
| #13 | | | Search: somatosensory tinnitus | 218 | 12:29:49 |
| #12 | | | Search: subjective tinnitus | 17,544 | 12:28:12 |
| #11 | | | Search: ear noise | 26,584 | 12:27:51 |
| #10 | | | Search: ear ringing | 17,590 | 12:27:34 |
| #9 | | | Search: tinnitus | 17,544 | 12:27:20 |
| #8 | | | Search: jaw disorders | 22,303 | 12:26:49 |
| #7 | | | Search: temporomandibular joint syndrome | 6,076 | 12:26:07 |
| #6 | | | Search: (craniomandibular disorder) AND (temporomandibular joint dysfunction) | 6,599 | 12:25:35 |
| #5 | | | Search: craniomandibular dysfunction | 772 | 12:23:46 |
| #4 | | | Search: cmd | 4,873 | 12:23:29 |
| #3 | | | Search: temporomandibular dysfunction | 11,879 | 12:23:19 |
| #2 | | | Search: tmd | 15,936 | 12:23:00 |
| #1 | | | Search: temporomandibular disorder | 22,689 | 12:22:50 |

Fig 4: Search protocol of the literature search in Medline (PubMed and PMC) (own illustration, 2024)

2. Fig. 5 below shows the first search protocol of the literature search in PEDro. The search was first carried out with the option 'Match all search terms' (AND), which did not lead to any results. This search protocol serves as a starting point for adapting the search strategy.

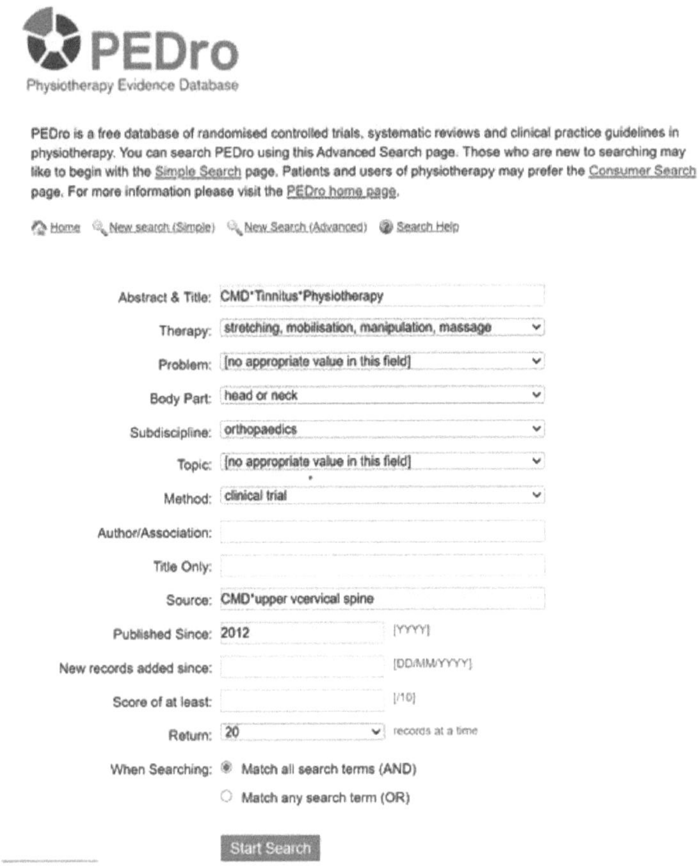


Fig 5: First search protocol of the literature search in PEDro with the option "Match all search terms" (AND). (Own illustration 2024)

3. Fig 6 below shows the second search protocol of the literature search in PEDro with the option "Match any search terms" (OR), which resulted in 264,751 hits and was recognised as a

This served as the basis for adapting the search strategy from Advanced Search to Simple Search.

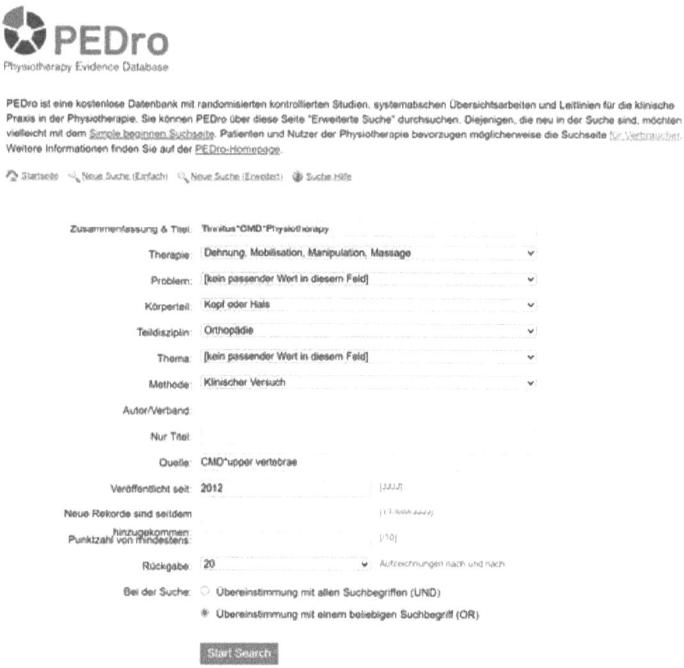


Fig 6: Second search protocol of the PEDro literature search with "Match any search terms" (OR). (own Presentation, 2024)

4 Fig. 7 below shows an overview of the "Simple search" in PEDro.

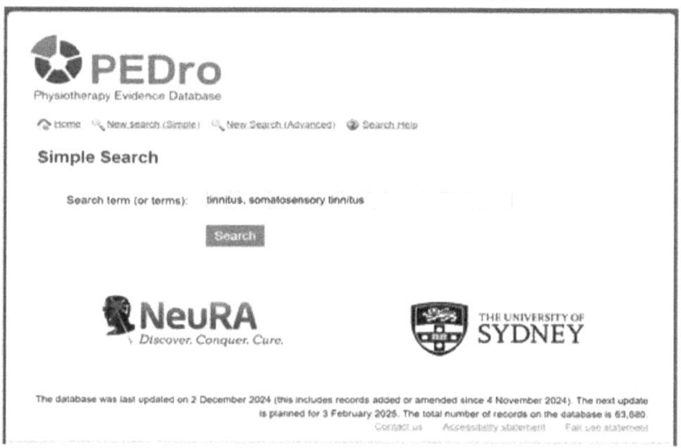


Fig 7: Third search protocol - overview of the "Simple search" in PEDro (own illustration 2024)

5. Fig. 8 below shows the final search protocol of the literature search in PEDro using "Simple Search", which resulted in 59 hits.

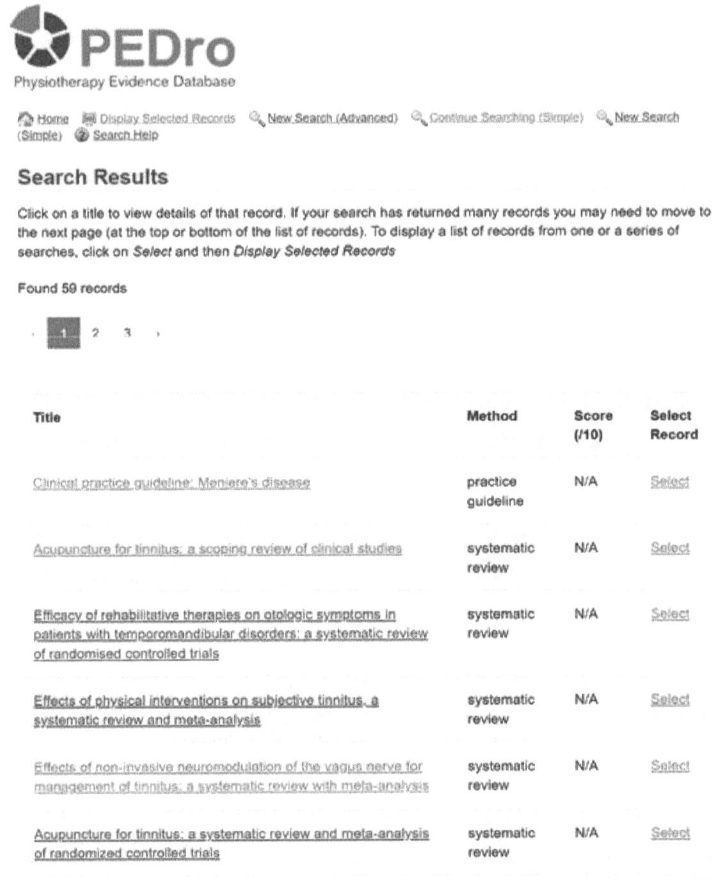

PEDro
Physiotherapy Evidence Database

Home | Display Selected Records | New Search (Advanced) | Continue Searching (Simple) | New Search (Simple) | Search Help

## Search Results

Click on a title to view details of that record. If your search has returned many records you may need to move to the next page (at the top or bottom of the list of records). To display a list of records from one or a series of searches, click on *Select* and then *Display Selected Records*

Found 59 records

‹ 1 2 3 ›

| Title | Method | Score (/10) | Select Record |
|---|---|---|---|
| Clinical practice guideline: Meniere's disease | practice guideline | N/A | Select |
| Acupuncture for tinnitus: a scoping review of clinical studies | systematic review | N/A | Select |
| Efficacy of rehabilitative therapies on otologic symptoms in patients with temporomandibular disorders: a systematic review of randomised controlled trials | systematic review | N/A | Select |
| Effects of physical interventions on subjective tinnitus, a systematic review and meta-analysis | systematic review | N/A | Select |
| Effects of non-invasive neuromodulation of the vagus nerve for management of tinnitus: a systematic review with meta-analysis | systematic review | N/A | Select |
| Acupuncture for tinnitus: a systematic review and meta-analysis of randomized controlled trials | systematic review | N/A | Select |

Fig 8: Final search protocol of the literature search in PEDro using "Simple Search". (own illustration, 2024)

6. Fig 9 below provides an overview of the "Advanced Search" in ScienceDirect

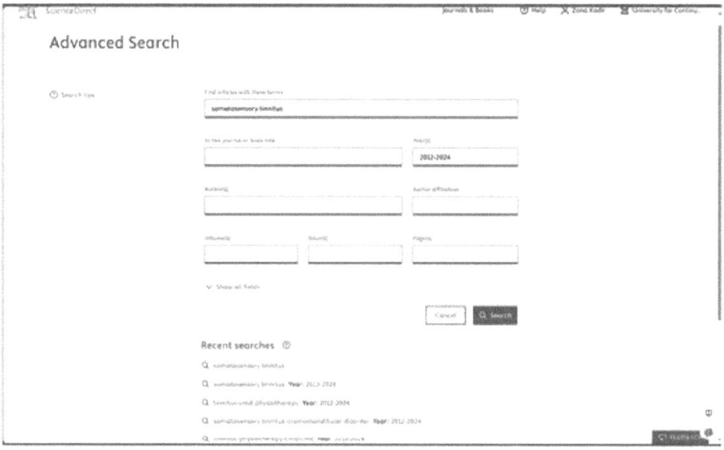


Fig 9: Overview of the "Advanced search" in ScienceDirect (own illustration 2024)

7. Fig. 10 below shows the first search log of the literature search in ScienceDirect with 999 hits.

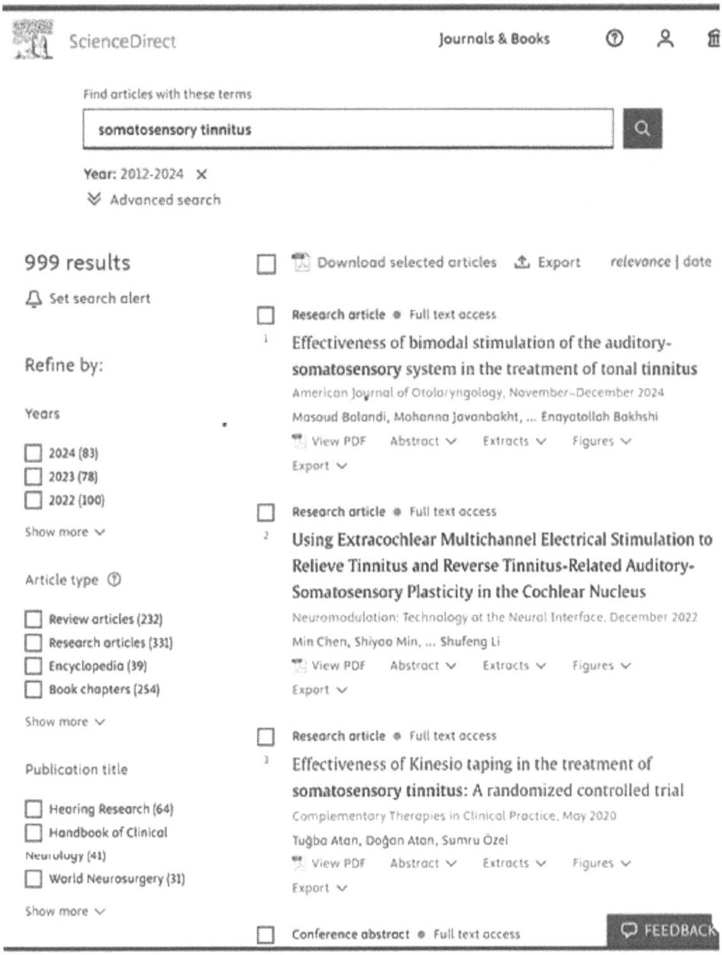


Fig 10: The first search protocol of the literature search in ScienceDirect (own illustration, 2024)

8. Fig. 11 below shows the final search protocol of the literature search after using the "Medicine and Dentistry" filter in ScienceDirect with 570 hits

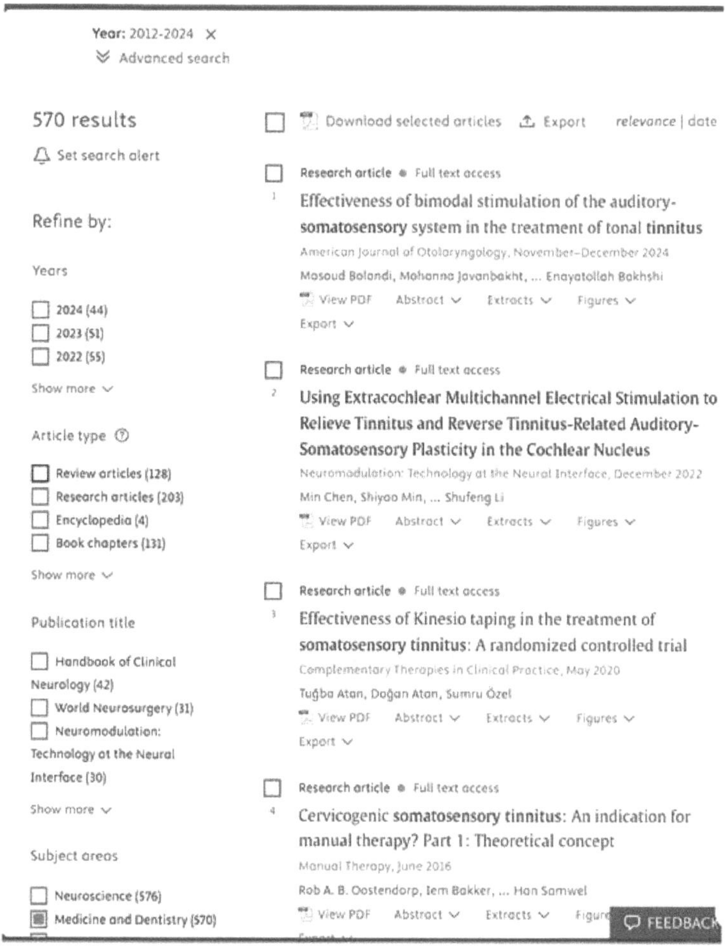


Fig 11: The final search protocol of the literature search in ScienceDirect (own illustration 2024)

Tab 20: CONSORT 2010 checklist for the study "Atan et. al., 2020", (own presentation 2024)

| Section/Topic | Number | Description of the | Completed information |
|---|---|---|---|
| **Title and Summary** | 1a | Identification in the title as a randomised study | Indicated in the title as a "randomised controlled trial". |
| | 1b | Structured summary of study design, methods, results and conclusions | Structured summary available in the introduction, describes study design, methods, results and conclusions. |
| **Introduction** | 2a | Scientific background and justification of the study | Background: The efficacy of kinesio taping for somatosensory tinnitus is unclear Aim: To evaluate the efficacy of KT in the context of somatosensory tinnitus. |
| | 2b | Precise question or hypotheses | Hypothesis: KT reduces the severity of somatosensory tinnitus better than sham tapping. |
| **Methods** | 3a | Description of the study design | Single-centre, prospective, randomised, sham-controlled, double-blind study with two groups (KT and ST). |
| | 3b | Important changes to the methods after the start of the programme | No changes reported. |
| | 4a | Suitability criteria of the test persons/patients | Patients with tinnitus for at least six weeks and neck complaints. Exclusion criteria: e.g. previous operations, middle ear diseases, pregnancy. |
| | 4b | Study environment and location | Medical Faculty of Hitit University, Department of Physical Medicine and Rehabilitation. |
| | 5 | Interventions carried out in each group | KT group: Kinesio taping on specific muscles. ST group (sham tape): Placebo taping without stretching. |
| | 6a | Fully defined primary and secondary endpoints | Primary endpoint: Tinnitus VAS. Secondary |
| | | | Endpoints: THI, cervical pain VAS, NDI. |
| | 6b | Changes in endpoints after the start of the study | No changes reported. |
| | 7a | How was the number of cases calculated? | Calculation with G-Power software; 15 patients per group based on minimal |

| | | | |
|---|---|---|---|
| | | | clinically important difference in VAS. |
| | 7b | Explanation of all interim analyses and termination criteria | No interim analyses or discontinuation criteria reported. |
| **Randomisation** | 8a | Method for generating the random allocation | Random allocation created by computer programme. |
| | 8b | Type of randomisation | Simple randomisation with sealed envelopes. |
| | 9 | Mechanisms for keeping the treatment sequence secret | Opaque, numbered envelopes used. |
| | 10 | Implementation of the randomisation | Independent researcher created allocation sequence; practitioners opened the envelopes. |
| | 11a | Who was allied? | Participants and outcome assessors were blinded. |
| | 11b | Description of the similarity of the interventions | Sham tapping was applied to the same muscles as in the ST group, but without stretching. |
| | 12a | Statistical methods for group comparison | Independent t-test for group comparisons; dependent t-test for before-after comparisons. |
| | 12b | Methods for additional analyses | No additional analyses reported. |
| **Results** | 13a | Number of randomised participants per group | KT group: 15, ST group: 15. |
| | 13b | Number of cancellations and reasons | Seven participants cancelled, reasons: Lack of time, transport problems. |
| | 14a | Recruitment and follow-up period | Recruitment to follow-up: 4 weeks. |
| | 14b | Why the study ended or was stopped | No premature termination. |
| | 15 | Patient characteristics at the start of the study | Table with demographic data and clinical characteristics in the article. |
| | 16 | Number of participants analysed | KT group: 15, ST group: 15, no deviations from randomisation. |
| | 17a | Results for endpoints and estimated effect sizes | Results in tables and figures with mean values and standard deviations. |
| | 17b | Binary endpoints | Not relevant. |
| | 18 | Additional analyses | No additional analyses were carried out. |

| | | | |
|---|---|---|---|
| | 19 | Damage | No harm or adverse effects reported. |
| **Discussion** | 20 | Study limitations | Small sample size, short Follow-up period, specific patient selection. |
| | 21 | Generalisability | Results apply to patients with somatosensory tinnitus and neck pain. |
| | 22 | Interpretation | KT effective for tinnitus, results consistent with previous studies. |
| **Other information** | 23 | Registration | ClinicalTrials.gov, NCT03782220. |
| | 24 | Protocol | Not reported. |
| | 25 | Financing | No funding received. |

Tab 21 : CONSORT 2010 checklist for the study "Aydogan et al., 2022", (own presentation 2024)

| Section/Topic | Number | Description of the | Completed information |
|---|---|---|---|
| **Title and Summary** | 1a | Identification in the title as a randomised study | Indicated as "randomised study" in the title. |
| | 1b | Structured summary of study design, methods, results and conclusions | Structured summary available, describes study design, methods, results and conclusions. |

| | | | |
|---|---|---|---|
| **Introduction** | 2a | Scientific background and justification of the study | Background: TENS could improve the symptoms of chronic subjective tinnitus. Aim: To investigate the efficacy of TENS therapy. |
| | 2b | Precise question or hypotheses | Hypothesis: TENS reduces the severity and effects of tinnitus better than education alone. |
| **Methods** | 3a | Description of the study design | Prospective, randomised, comparative study with two groups (TENS group and control group). |
| | 3b | Important changes to the methods after the start of the programme | No changes reported. |
| | 4a | Eligibility criteria of the test subjects/patients | Patients with chronic subjective tinnitus, normal hearing, without neurological or psychiatric disorders. Exclusion: Pacemaker, previous ear surgery. |
| | 4b | Study environment and location | Ankara University Faculty of Medicine, Audiology Department. |
| | 5 | Interventions carried out in each Group | Study group (TENS): 20 sessions of TENS therapy. Control group: Only education about tinnitus. |
| | 6a | Fully defined primary and secondary endpoints | Primary endpoint: tinnitus severity. Secondary endpoints: VAS loudness, THI, SF-36. |
| | 6b | Changes in endpoints after the start of the study | No changes reported. |
| | 7a | How was the number of cases calculated? | Calculation with G*Power software; 23 participants per group based on expected effect sizes. |
| | 7b | Explanation of all interim analyses and termination criteria | No interim analyses or discontinuation criteria reported. |
| **Randomisation** | 8a | Method for generating the random allocation | Random allocation created by computer programme. |
| | 8b | Type of randomisation | Simple randomisation. |
| | 9 | Mechanisms for keeping the treatment sequence secret | Mechanism for confidentiality not explicitly described. |
| | 10 | Implementation of the | No specific details on |

| | | | |
|---|---|---|---|
| | | randomisation | implementation reported. |
| | 11a | Who was blinded? | Allocation of participants and outcome assessment not mentioned; practitioners were not blinded. |
| | 11b | Description of the similarity of the interventions | Control group received no intervention, only education. |
| | 12a | Statistical methods for group comparison | t-tests and Mann-Whitney U-test for group comparisons; paired t-tests for before and after comparisons. |
| | 12b | Methods for additional analyses | No additional analyses reported. |
| **Results** | 13a | Number of randomised participants per group | TENS group: 23, control group: 23. |
| | 13b | Number of cancellations and reasons | No reported failures. |
| | 14a | Recruitment and follow-up period | Recruitment to follow-up: March 2020 to December 2021. |
| | 14b | Why the study ended or was stopped | No premature termination. |
| | 15 | Patient characteristics at the start of the study | Table with demographic data and clinical characteristics in the article. |
| | 16 | Number of participants analysed | TENS group: 23, control group: 23, no deviations from randomisation. |
| | 17a | Results for endpoints and estimated effect sizes | Results presented in tables with mean values and standard deviations. |
| | 17b | Binary endpoints | Not relevant. |
| | 18 | Additional analyses | No additional analyses performed. |
| | 19 | Damage | No harm or adverse effects reported. |
| **Discussion** | 20 | Study limitations | No blinding of the practitioners, heterogeneous participant characteristics, short<br>Follow-up period. |
| | 21 | Generalisability | Results apply to patients with chronic subjective tinnitus. |
| | 22 | Interpretation | TENS effective for tinnitus, results consistent with previous studies. |
| **Other information** | 23 | Registration | ClinicalTrials.gov, NCTXXXX. |
| | 24 | Protocol | Not reported. |

| | | | |
|---|---|---|---|
| | 25 | Financing | No funding received. |

Tab 22: CONSORT 2010 checklist for the study "Delgado de la Serna et. al., 2020", (own Presentation 2024)

| Section/Topic | Number | Description of the | Completed information |
|---|---|---|---|
| **Title and Summary** | 1a | Identification in the title as a randomised study | Indicated in the title as "randomised clinical trial". |
| | 1b | Structured summary of study design, methods, results and conclusions | Structured summary available, describes study design, methods, results and conclusions. |
| **Introduction** | 2a | Scientific background and justification of the study | Background: CMD is associated with tinnitus; Manual therapy could improve these symptoms. Aim: Comparison of movement/education alone vs. Movement/Education + MT. |
| | 2b | Precise question or hypotheses | Hypothesis: Additional manual therapy significantly improves clinical, psychological and physical outcomes. |
| **Methods** | 3a | Description of the study design | Multicentre, randomised, parallel-group clinical trial. |
| | 3b | Important changes to the methods after the start of the programme | No changes reported. |
| | 4a | Eligibility criteria of the test subjects/patients | Patients with CMD-associated tinnitus, age 18-65 years. Exclusion: |
| | | | ENT pathologies, neurological diseases, previous CMD treatment. |
| | 4b | Study environment and location | Three private physiotherapy clinics in Spain. |
| | 5 | Interventions carried out in each group | Study group: movement/education + manual therapy. Control group: movement/education alone. |
| | 6a | Fully defined primary and secondary endpoints | Primary: CMD pain (NPRS), tinnitus severity (VAS). Secondary: THI, CF-PDI, SF-12, BDI-II, PPT, mandibular range of motion. |
| | 6b | Changes in endpoints after the start of the study | No changes reported. |

| | | | |
|---|---|---|---|
| | 7a | How was the number of cases calculated? | Calculation based on expected differences in VAS; target: 30 participants per group. |
| | 7b | Explanation of all interim analyses and cancellation criteria | No interim analyses or discontinuation criteria reported. |
| **Randomisation** | 8a | Method for generating the random allocation | Computer-generated random numbers. |
| | 8b | Type of randomisation | Simple randomisation; concealed allocation with sealed envelopes. |
| | 9 | Mechanisms for keeping the treatment sequence secret | Concealed allocation ensured by sealed envelopes. |
| | 10 | Implementation of the randomisation | External researcher performed randomisation; group allocation by blinded reviewer. |
| | 11a | Who was blinded? | Outcome assessment was blinded; patients may not have been completely blinded. |
| | 11b | Description of the similarity of the interventions | Both groups received similar exercise and education; manual therapy was added to the study group. |
| | 12a | Statistical methods for group comparison | ANCOVA analyses with covariates (e.g. sex); Bonferroni |
| | | | Correction for multiple comparisons. |
| | 12b | Methods for additional analyses | No additional analyses reported. |
| **Results** | 13a | Number of randomised participants per group | Study group: 31, control group: 30. |
| | 13b | Number of cancellations and reasons | No failures reported. |
| | 14a | Recruitment and follow-up period | January to December 2017; follow-up up to six months after the intervention. |
| | 14b | Why the study ended or was stopped | Regular end; no premature termination. |
| | 15 | Patient characteristics at the start of the study | Table with demographic data and clinical characteristics in the article. |
| | 16 | Number of participants analysed | Study group: 31, control group: 30, no deviations from randomisation. |

| | | | |
|---|---|---|---|
| | 17a | Results for endpoints and estimated effect sizes | Results presented in tables with mean values and standard deviations. |
| | 17b | Binary endpoints | Not relevant. |
| | 18 | Additional analyses | No additional analyses performed. |
| | 19 | Damage | No harm or adverse effects reported. |
| **Discussion** | 20 | Study limitations | No control group without intervention; potential placebo effect not investigated; no objective diagnostic methods for tinnitus. |
| | 21 | Generalisability | Results apply to CMD-associated tinnitus in patients in the age group 18-65 years. |
| | 22 | Interpretation | Results show the superiority of exercise/education + MT over exercise/education alone. |
| **Other information** | 23 | Registration | ClinicalTrials.gov, NCT02850055. |
| | 24 | Protocol | Not reported. |
| | 25 | Financing | No funding received. |

Tab 23: CONSORT 2010 checklist for the study "Eladl et. al., 2022", (own presentation 2024)

| Section/Topic | Number | Description of the | Completed information |
|---|---|---|---|
| **Title and Summary** | 1a | Identification in the title as a randomised study | Indicated in the title as a "randomised controlled trial". |
| | 1b | Structured summary of study design, methods, results and conclusions | Structured summary available, describes study design, methods, results and conclusions. |
| **Introduction** | 2a | Scientific background and justification of the study | Background: OST is influenced by physical movement. Aim: To investigate PBMT and physiotherapy exercises. |
| | 2b | Precise question or hypotheses | Hypothesis: PBMT in combination with exercises improves tinnitus and ROM significantly better than PBMT alone. |
| **Methods** | 3a | Description of the study design | Randomised, double-blind, controlled study with two groups (PBMT+therapy vs. PBMT alone). |
| | 3b | Important changes to the | No changes reported. |

| | | | |
|---|---|---|---|
| | | methods after the start of the programme | |
| | 4a | Suitability of the test subjects/patients | Patients with CST (45-55 years), stable symptoms for at least 3 months. Exclusion: neurological/ontological diseases. |
| | 4b | Study environment and location | Faculty of Physiotherapy, Cairo University. |
| | 5 | Interventions carried out in each Group | Group A: PBMT + exercise programme; Group B: PBMT alone. |
| | 6a | Fully defined primary and secondary endpoints | Primary: VAS for tinnitus. Secondary: THI, ROM of the cervical spine. |
| | 6b | Changes in endpoints after the start of the study | No changes reported. |
| | 7a | How was the number of cases calculated? | Calculated with G*Power: 20 participants per group (incl. dropout rate). |
| | 7b | Explanation of all interim analyses and termination criteria | No interim analyses or discontinuation criteria reported. |
| **Randomisation** | 8a | Method for generating the random allocation | Computer-generated block randomisation (block size 4). |
| | 8b | Type of randomisation | Egg after randomisation with concealed allocation. |
| | 9 | Mechanisms for keeping the treatment sequence secret | Sealed, numbered, opaque envelopes. |
| | 10 | Implementation of the randomisation | Randomisation performed by independent researcher. |
| | 11a | Who was allied? | Patients and result evaluators; practitioners are not allied. |
| | 11b | Description of the similarity of the interventions | PBMT protocol identical in both groups; group A received additional exercises. |
| | 12a | Statistical methods for group comparison | Mixed design MANOVA for Time and Group interactions; Bonferroni correction. |
| | 12b | Methods for additional analyses | No additional analyses reported. |
| **Results** | 13a | Number of randomised participants per group | Group A: 20, Group B: 20. |
| | 13b | Number of cancellations and reasons | No reported failures. |

| | | | |
|---|---|---|---|
| | 14a | Recruitment and follow-up period | Recruitment: December 2018 to April 2019;<br>Follow-up: 8 weeks. |
| | 14b | Why the study ended or was stopped | No premature termination. |
| | 15 | Patient characteristics at the start of the study | Age and<br>Gender distribution similar in both groups (see table). |
| | 16 | Number of participants analysed | All 40 randomised participants were analysed. |
| | 17a | Results for endpoints and estimated effect sizes | Significant differences in favour of group A for VAS, THI and ROM. |
| | 17b | Binary endpoints | Not relevant. |
| | 18 | Additional analyses | No additional analyses performed. |
| | 19 | Damage | No reported adverse events. |
| **Discussion** | 20 | Study limitations | No long-term follow-up; no control group without intervention; no placebo comparison. |
| | 21 | Generalisability | Results apply to CST patients aged 4555 years. |
| | 22 | Interpretation | PBMT + exercise more effective than PBMT alone; results consistent with previous studies. |
| **Other information** | 23 | Registration | ClinicalTrials.gov, NCT0464115. |
| | 24 | Protocol | Not reported. |
| | 25 | Financing | Funded by Princess Nourah bint Abdulrahman University Researchers Supporting Project. |

Tab 24: CONSORT 2010 checklist for the study "Fobbe et al., 2022", (own presentation 2024)

| **Section/Topic** | **Number** | **Description of the** | **Completed information** |
|---|---|---|---|
| **Title and Summary** | 1a | Identification in the title as a randomised study | Indicated in the title as a "prospective randomised study". |
| | 1b | Structured<br>Summary of study design, methods, results and conclusions | Structured summary available, describes study design, methods, results and conclusions. |
| **Introduction** | 2a | Scientific background and justification of the study | Background: Relationship between muscular tension and tinnitus investigated.<br>Aim: Effectiveness of manual therapy. |

| | | | |
|---|---|---|---|
| | 2b | Precise question or hypotheses | Hypothesis: Manual therapy significantly improves tinnitus and vertigo symptoms. |
| **Methods** | 3a | Description of the study design | Prospective, randomised clinical trial. |
| | 3b | Important changes to the methods after the start of the programme | No changes reported. |
| | 4a | Suitability of the test subjects/patients | Adults with tinnitus and cervical spine complaints, without operations or injuries to the neck or ear. |
| | 4b | Study environment and location | Hannover Medical School, Germany. |
| | 5 | Interventions carried out in each group | Intervention group: Manual therapy; Control group: waiting list. |
| | 6a | Fully defined primary and secondary endpoints | Primary endpoints: THI and DHI; secondary endpoint: change in muscle tone. |
| | 6b | Changes in endpoints after the start of the study | No changes reported. |
| | 7a | How was the number of cases calculated? | Calculated with G*Power: 40 participants per group, taking dropouts into account. |
| | 7b | Explanation of all interim analyses and cancellation conditions | No interim analyses or discontinuation criteria reported. |
| **Randomisation** | 8a | Method for generating the random allocation | Random allocation through sealed envelopes. |
| | 8b | Type of randomisation | Block randomisation (1:1). |
| | 9 | Mechanisms for keeping the treatment sequence secret | Sealed, numbered, opaque envelopes. |
| | 10 | Implementation of the randomisation | Randomisation carried out by independent employees. |
| | 11a | Who was allied? | Allocation of physiotherapists; participants and investigators were not blinded. |
| | 11b | Description of the similarity of the interventions | Intervention group received manual therapy, control group waited. |
| | 12a | Statistical methods for group comparison | Mann-Whitney U test and Wilcoxon test for group and time comparisons. |

| | | | |
|---|---|---|---|
| | 12b | Methods for additional analyses | No additional analyses reported. |
| **Results** | 13a | Number of randomised participants per group | Intervention group: 37, control group: 33. |
| | 13b | Number of cancellations and reasons | Dropouts due to the corona pandemic (fear of infection). |
| | 14a | Recruitment and follow-up period | Recruitment: May 2020 to February 2021;<br>Follow-up: 6 weeks. |
| | 14b | Why the study ended or was stopped | Scheduled end of the study. |
| | 15 | Patient characteristics at the start of the study | groups were similar in age, gender, duration and localisation of tinnitus. |
| | 16 | Number of participants analysed | Intervention group: 37, control group: 33. |
| | 17a | Results for endpoints and estimated effect sizes | Significant improvement in THI and DHI in the intervention group. |
| | 17b | Binary endpoints | Not relevant. |
| | 18 | Additional analyses | No additional analyses performed. |
| | 19 | Damage | No reported adverse events. |
| **Discussion** | 20 | Study limitations | Lack of placebo control group, lack of blinding of participants and investigators. |
| | 21 | Generalisability | Results apply to patients with CST and cervical spine complaints. |
| | 22 | Interpretation | Manual therapy effective for CST and associated complaints. |
| **Other information** | 23 | Registration | Ethics Committee MHH, No. 9111 BOS 2020. |
| | 24 | Protocol | Not reported. |
| | 25 | Financing | Open Access Funding through Project DEAL. |

Tab 25: CONSORT 2010 checklist for the study "Michiels et al., 2016",(own illustration 2024)

| Section/Topic | Number | Description of the | Completed information |
|---|---|---|---|
| **Title and Summary** | 1a | Identification in the title as a randomised study | Indicated in the title as a "randomised controlled trial". |
| | 1b | Structured Summary of study design, | Structured summary available. Describes design, methods, |

| | | | |
|---|---|---|---|
| | | Methods, results and conclusions | Results and conclusions. |
| **Introduction** | 2a | Scientific background and justification of the study | Background: Connection between the cervical spine and tinnitus. Objective: Effect of cervical physiotherapy. |
| | 2b | Precise question or hypotheses | Hypothesis: Cervical physiotherapy reduces subjective tinnitus complaints in CST patients. |
| **Methods** | 3a | Description of the study design | Randomised, controlled study with delayed start. |
| | 3b | Important changes to the methods after the start of the programme | No changes reported. |
| | 4a | Suitability of the test subjects/patients | Adults with chronic tinnitus (TFI: 25-90), NBQ >14, no objective causes of tinnitus. |
| | 4b | Study environment and location | University Hospital Antwerp, tertiary tinnitus clinic. |
| | 5 | Interventions carried out in each group | Immediate start group: Physiotherapy for 6 weeks. Delayed start group: waiting list, then physiotherapy. |
| | 6a | Fully defined primary and secondary endpoints | Primary endpoint: TFI. Secondary endpoints: NBQ, GPE. |
| | 6b | Changes in endpoints after the start of the study | No changes reported. |
| | 7a | How was the number of cases calculated? | Calculation based on pilot data, target: 40 participants. |
| | 7b | Explanation of all interim analyses and termination criteria | No interim analyses or discontinuation criteria reported. |
| **Randomisation** | 8a | Method for generating the random allocation | Block randomisation with variable block lengths. |
| | 8b | Type of randomisation | Random numbers generated with Microsoft Excel. |
| | 9 | Mechanisms for keeping the treatment sequence secret | Concealed randomisation list is used. |
| | 10 | Implementation of the randomisation | Randomisation performed according to output measurements. |
| | 11a | Who was allied? | Alliance of the therapists and the examiner. |
| | 11b | Description of the similarity of the interventions | The control group received cervical physiotherapy after a |

| | | | |
|---|---|---|---|
| | | | waiting period. |
| | 12a | Statistical methods for group comparison | Two-way ANOVA, t-tests, chi-square tests. |
| | 12b | Methods for additional analyses | No additional analyses reported. |
| **Results** | 13a | Number of randomised participants per group | Immediate start group: 19, delayed start group: 19. |
| | 13b | Number of cancellations and reasons | Two patients refused treatment after randomisation. |
| | 14a | Recruitment and follow-up period | Recruitment and follow-up: one year. |
| | 14b | Why the study ended or was stopped | Scheduled end after study period. |
| | 15 | Patient characteristics at the start of the study | Table with demographic and clinical data available. |
| | 16 | Number of participants analysed | Immediate start group: 19, delayed start group: 19. |
| | 17a | Results for endpoints and estimated effect sizes | TFI: Significant improvement after treatment. |
| | 17b | Binary endpoints | GPE: 53% improvement after treatment, 24% after follow-up. |
| | 18 | Additional analyses | No additional analyses were carried out. |
| | 19 | Damage | No adverse events reported. |
| **Discussion** | 20 | Study limitations | Limited Sample size, no placebo control group, short follow-up. |
| | 21 | Generalisability | Results apply to CST patients. |
| | 22 | Interpretation | Physiotherapy effective for CST. Further research recommended. |
| **Other information** | 23 | Registration | ClinicalTrials.gov, NCT02016313. |
| | 24 | Protocol | Protocol not reported. |
| | 25 | Financing | Research grant from the University of Antwerp. |

Tab 26: COSORT 2010 checklist for the "Plaza- Monzano et.al.,2022" study (own presentation 2024)

| **Section/Topic** | **Number** | **Description of the** | **Completed information** |
|---|---|---|---|
| **Title and Summary** | | | |
| **Labelling in the title** | 1a | Identification in the title as a randomised study | The title clearly indicates that this is a randomised clinical trial. |
| **Structured Summary** | 1b | Structured summary of the study design, | Summary includes study design, interventions, |

| | | | |
|---|---|---|---|
| | | methods, results and Conclusions | endpoints and main results. |
| **Introduction** | | | |
| **Background and goals** | 2a | Scientific background and justification of the study | Aim: This study investigates the influence of clinical, psychological and psychophysical variables on the treatment outcomes of tinnitus associated with TMD. |
| **Research question or hypotheses** | 2b | Precise question or hypotheses | Hypothesis: Higher tinnitus severity at the start of the study predicts better treatment results. |
| **Methods** | | | |
| **Study design** | 3a | Description of the study design (e.g. parallel, factorial), including allocation ratio | Parallel group RCT with 1:1 randomisation. |
| **Changes to the methods** | 3b | Important changes to the methods after the start of the programme with reasons | No changes reported. |
| **Test subjects/patients** | 4a | Eligibility criteria of the test subjects/patients | Included: TMD-associated tinnitus, age 18-65 years. Excluded: Neurological pathologies, previous physiotherapy. |
| **Surroundings and location** | 4b | Study environment and location | Location University Hospital Antwerp, Belgium |
| **Intervention/treatment** | 5 | Interventions carried out in each group with precise details | Expehmental group: manual therapy + exercises + education. Control group: exercises + education. |
| **Endpoints** | 6a | Fully defined primary and secondary endpoints | Primary: Tinnitus severity (VAS), tinnitus handicap (THI). Secondary: Pressure pain thresholds (PPT), depression level (BDI-II). |
| **Changes to the end points** | 6b | Changes in endpoints after the start of the study with reasons | No changes reported. |
| **Determination of case numbers** | 7a | How was the number of cases calculated? | Based on expected changes in tinnitus severity at 6-month follow-up. |

| | | | |
|---|---|---|---|
| **Interim analyses** | 7b | If applicable, explanation of all interim analyses and cancellation | No interim analyses or discontinuation criteria reported. |
| **Randomisation** | | | |
| **Generation of the Treatment sequence** | 8a | Method for generating the random allocation | Block randomisation with hidden list. |
| **Type of randomisation** | 8b | Type of randomisation; details of any restrictions | Block formation, variable block size. |
| **Confidentiality of the treatment sequence** | 9 | Mechanisms for keeping the allocation sequence secret | Hidden randomisation lists are used. |
| **Realisation** | 10 | Who carried out the randomisation and who allocated the participants to the interventions | Random allocation by study director; Interventions by therapists. |
| **Alliance** | 11a | If conducted, who was involved? (e.g. participants, doctors, therapists) | Investigators and therapists were blinded, participants were not. |
| **Similarity of the interventions** | 11b | If relevant, Description of the similarity of the interventions | Exercises and education in both groups similar; manual therapy only in the experimental group. |
| **Statistical methods** | | | |
| **Comparison of the groups** | 12a | Statistical methods for comparing the groups with regard to primary and secondary endpoints | Multivariate Regression models; significance level $p < 0.05$. |
| **Additional analyses** | 12b | Methods for subgroup analyses, adjusted analyses | Hierarchical regression analyses were performed. |
| **Results** | | | |
| **Participant flow** | 13a | Number of study participants randomly assigned and analysed | 61 participants randomised; 56 in the final analysis. |
| **Exclusions** | 13b | Number of Study dropouts and exclusions after randomisation | 5 participants dropped out (reasons documented). |
| **Admission/recruitment** | 14a | Recruitment and follow-up period | Recruitment over 12 months, follow-up up to 6 months. |
| **End of study** | 14b | Why the study ended or was stopped | Planned end after completion of the follow-up observations. |

| | | | |
|---|---|---|---|
| **Patient characteristics at the start of the study** | 15 | Demographic and clinical characteristics for each group | Baseline data comparable between groups; no significant differences. |
| **Number of patients analysed** | 16 | Number of participants in the analysis and comparison with the original allocation | 56 of 61 included participants analysed; corresponds to 92 % retention rate. |
| **Results and estimation methods** | 17a | Results for primary and secondary endpoints | Significant improvements in tinnitus severity and handicap in the experimental group. |
| **Effect sizes** | 17b | Absolute and relative effect sizes | Effect sizes reported for VAS and THI; relative improvements shown. |
| **Additional analyses** | 18 | Results of subgroup analyses and adjusted Analyses | Subgroup analyses were performed for gender and baseline values. |
| **Damage** | 19 | Important damage (undesirable effects) | No serious adverse events reported. |
| **Discussion** | | | |
| **Limitations** | 20 | Study limitations and potential biases | Small sample; no long-term data beyond 6 months. |
| **Generalisability** | 21 | Generalisability (external validity, applicability) of the study results | Results applicable to similar populations with TMD-associated tinnitus. |
| **Interpretation** | 22 | Interpretation consistent with results, weighing up the benefits and harms | Results support the use of manual therapy for TMD-associated tinnitus. |
| **Other information** | | | |
| **Registration** | 23 | Registration number and name of the study registry | ClinicalTrials.gov: NCT02850055 |
| **Protocol** | 24 | Where the complete minutes can be viewed | Protocol available on request. |
| **Financing** | 25 | Sources of funding and other support | Funded by university scholarship; no conflicts of interest reported. |

Tab 27: CONSORT 2010 checklist for the study "Tutar et.al.,2020", (own presentation 2024)

| Section/Topic | Number | Description of the | Completed information |
|---|---|---|---|
| **Title and Summary** | **1a** | Identification in the title as a randomised study | Indicated in the title as a "randomised controlled trial". |
| | **1b** | Structured Summary of study design, methods, results and | Structured summary available, describes design, methods and |

| | | | |
|---|---|---|---|
| | | conclusions | results. |
| **Introduction** | **2a** | Scientific background and justification of the study | Background: TENS was investigated as a potential therapy for tinnitus. |
| | **2b** | Precise question or hypotheses | Hypothesis: TENS reduces subjective tinnitus complaints and improves quality of life. |
| **Methods** | **3a** | Description of the study design | Prospective, randomised, placebo-controlled study with three groups. |
| | **3b** | Important changes to the methods after the start of the programme | No changes reported. |
| | **4a** | Suitability of the test subjects/patients | Patients with chronic subjective tinnitus (>3 months), age: 18-65 years. |
| | **4b** | Study environment and location | Clinic in Turkey, prospective study. |
| | **5** | Interventions carried out in each Group | Group A: TENS on one ear; group B: TENS on both ears; group C: placebo. |
| | **6a** | Fully defined primary and secondary endpoints | Primary: THI. Secondary: DASS. |
| | **6b** | Changes in endpoints after the start of the study | No changes reported. |
| | **7a** | How was the number of cases calculated? | Case number of 60 patients was based on previous studies on TENS and tinnitus. |
| | **7b** | Explanation of all interim analyses and cancellation conditions | No interim analyses or discontinuation criteria reported. |
| **Randomisation** | **8a** | Method for generating the random allocation | Computerised randomisation using a random generator. |
| | **8b** | Type of randomisation | Random allocation without restrictions. |
| | **9** | Mechanisms for keeping the treatment sequence secret | Sealed envelopes to ensure blinding. |
| | **10** | Implementation of the randomisation | Randomisation by an independent researcher after recruitment. |
| | **11a** | Who was allied? | Subjects blinded; treating physicians not blinded. |
| | **11b** | Description of the similarity of the interventions | Placebo group received no electrical stimulation, |

| | | | |
|---|---|---|---|
| | | | otherwise identical conditions. |
| | **12a** | Statistical methods for group comparison | One-way ANOVA, post hoc Tukey tests. |
| | **12b** | Methods for additional analyses | No additional analyses performed. |
| **Results** | **13a** | Number of randomised participants per group | Group A: 20, Group B: 20, Group C: 20. |
| | **13b** | Number of cancellations and reasons | No dropouts reported. |
| | **14a** | Recruitment and follow-up period | Recruitment and follow-up: January-December 2018. |
| | **14b** | Why the study ended or was stopped | Scheduled end after study period. |
| | **15** | Patient characteristics at the start of the study | Table with demographic and clinical data available. |
| | **16** | Number of participants analysed | All 60 randomised participants were analysed. |
| | **17a** | Results for endpoints and estimated effect sizes | THI score: Significant Improvement in groups A and B. |
| | **17b** | Binary endpoints | Responder rate based on THI >10 points improvement. |
| | **18** | Additional analyses | No additional analyses performed. |
| | **19** | Damage | No adverse events reported. |
| **Discussion** | **20** | Study limitations | No long-term data, lack of double blinding, small sample size. |
| | **21** | Generalisability | Results possibly limited to similar populations. |
| | **22** | Interpretation | TENS has therapeutic effect and placebo effect, further research necessary. |
| **Other information** | **23** | Registration | Not reported. |
| | **24** | Protocol | Protocol not available. |
| | **25** | Financing | No funding reported. |

Tab 28: CONSORT 2010 checklist for the "Van der Wal et al., 2020" study (own presentation 2024)

| **Section/Topic** | **Number** | **Description of the** | **Completed information** |
|---|---|---|---|
| **Title and Summary** | **1a** | Identification in the title as a randomised study | Indicated in the title as a "randomised controlled trial". |
| | **1b** | Structured Summary of study design, | Structured summary available, describes |

| | | | |
|---|---|---|---|
| | | Methods, results and conclusions | Design, methods and results. |
| **Introduction** | **2a** | Scientific background and justification of the study | Background: Relationship between TMD and tinnitus investigated. |
| | **2b** | Precise question or hypotheses | Hypothesis: Orofacial treatment reduces tinnitus complaints. |
| **Methods** | **3a** | Description of the study design | Randomised controlled trial with delayed treatment design. |
| | **3b** | Important changes to the methods after the start of the programme | No changes reported. |
| | **4a** | Eligibility criteria of the test subjects/patients | Patients with TMD and moderate to severe tinnitus (TFI 25-90 points). |
| | **4b** | Study environment and location | Tertiary Tinnitus Clinic, University Hospital Antwerp, Belgium. |
| | **5** | Interventions carried out in each<br>Group | Early start group: Immediate treatment;<br>Delayed start group: treatment after 9 weeks. |
| | **6a** | Fully defined primary and secondary endpoints | Primary: TQ. Secondary: TFI. |
| | **6b** | Changes in endpoints after the start of the study | No changes reported. |
| | **7a** | How was the number of cases calculated? | Based on 80% power and 8.72 points as clinically relevant change in TQ. |
| | **7b** | Explanation of all interim analyses and termination criteria | No interim analyses or discontinuation criteria reported. |
| **Randomisation** | **8a** | Method for generating the random allocation | Block randomisation with variable block length, generated in Excel. |
| | **8b** | Type of randomisation | Random 1:1 assignment. |
| | **9** | Mechanisms for keeping the treatment sequence secret | Concealed randomisation by independent list. |
| | **10** | Implementation of the randomisation | Independent researcher after baseline measurements. |
| | **11a** | Who was blinded? | Practitioner blinded;<br>Patients not blinded. |
| | **11b** | Description of the similarity of the interventions | Same treatment in both groups after the delay period. |
| | **12a** | Statistical methods for | Mann-Whitney U-test, |

| | | | |
|---|---|---|---|
| | | group comparison | independent t-test. |
| | **12b** | Methods for additional analyses | Additional analyses on the clinical relevance of TQ and TFI. |
| **Results** | **13a** | Number of randomised participants per group | Early start group: 40, delayed start group: 40. |
| | **13b** | Number of cancellations and reasons | Early start group: 3 dropouts; Delayed start group: 2 dropouts. |
| | **14a** | Recruitment and follow-up period | January 2017 to December 2018. |
| | **14b** | Why the study ended or was stopped | Scheduled end after study period. |
| | **15** | Patient characteristics at the start of the study | Table with demographic and clinical data available. |
| | **16** | Number of participants analysed | Early start group: 37, delayed start group: 38. |
| | **17a** | Results for endpoints and estimated effect sizes | Significant improvements in TFI in both groups. |
| | **17b** | Binary endpoints | Proportion of patients with clinically relevant improvements reported. |
| | **18** | Additional analyses | No further analyses reported. |
| | **19** | Damage | No adverse events reported. |
| **Discussion** | **20** | Study limitations | No comparison group, lag design limited informative value. |
| | **21** | Generalisability | Results apply to tertiary Tinnitus populations. |
| | **22** | Interpretation | Orofacial treatment reduced Tinnitus complaints, further studies necessary. |
| **Other information** | **23** | Registration | ClinicalTrials.gov, NCT03209297. |
| | **24** | Protocol | Published. |
| | **25** | Financing | Research grant from Fonds voor wetenschappelijk |
| | | | onderzoek Vlaanderen (FWO). |

Tab 29: CONSORT 2010 checklist for the study "Zhe Yu et.al.,2024",(own illustration 2024)

| Section/Topic | Number | Description of the | Recording in the study |
|---|---|---|---|
| **Title and Summary** | | | |
| **Title and Summary** | 1a | Identification in the title as a randomised study | Yes, the title describes the study as randomised. |

| | | | |
|---|---|---|---|
| | 1b | Structured summary of study design, methods, results and conclusions | Yes, the Summary is structured and summarises the most important aspects of the study. |
| **Introduction** | | | |
| **Background and goals** | 2a | Scientific background and justification of the study | Detailed description, especially on the pathogenesis of somatosensory tinnitus. |
| | 2b | Precise question or hypotheses | Yes, the question and the objective are clearly defined. |
| **Methods** | | | |
| **Study design** | 3a | Description of the study design, including allocation ratio | Randomised controlled trial with immediate and late start groups (1:1 ratio). |
| | 3b | Important changes to the methods after the start of the programme with reasons | No changes indicated. |
| **Test subjects/patients** | 4a | Eligibility criteria of the test subjects/patients | Clearly defined, including inclusion and exclusion criteria. |
| | 4b | Study environment and location | Conducted at the hospital of Fudan University. |
| **Intervention/treatment** | 5 | Interventions carried out in each group with details | Physiotherapy with a detailed description of the exercises. |
| **End points** | 6a | Fully defined primary and secondary endpoints | VAS, THI and NPRS clearly defined as main endpoints. |
| | 6b | Changes to the endpoints after | No changes reported. |
| | | Start of study with reasons | |
| **Determination of case numbers** | 7a | How was the number of cases calculated? | Not specified. |
| | 7b | Interim analyses and Cancellation criteria | Not relevant. |
| **Randomisation** | | | |
| **Generation of the Treatment sequence** | 8a | Method for generating the random allocation | Computer-generated randomisation. |
| | 8b | Type of randomisation; details of any restrictions | No restrictions specified. |
| **Mechanisms for keeping the treatment sequence** | 9 | Mechanisms for implementing the | Concealed allocation by an external researcher. |

| | | | |
|---|---|---|---|
| **secret** | | allocation sequence | |
| **Realisation** | 10 | Who carried out the random allocation, who accepted participants? | External researcher carried out the randomisation. |
| **Alliance** | 11a | If carried out, who was allied? | Assessors were allied. Subjects not allied |
| | 11b | Description of the similarity of the interventions | Not applicable, as no placebo group. |
| **Statistical methods** | 12a | Statistical methods for primary and secondary endpoints | T-tests and Mann-Whitney U-tests. |
| | 12b | Methods for additional analyses | Regressions for the identification of prognostic indicators. |
| **Results** | | | |
| **Inclusions and exclusions** | 13a | Number of study participants in each group | Yes, stated (n = 43; immediate start: n = 20, late start: n = 23). |
| | 13b | Number of students dropping out with reasons | Yes, three participants could not be contacted. |
| **Admission/recruitment** | 14a | Recruitment and follow-up period | February to May 2019. |
| | 14b | Why the study ended or was stopped | Not applicable. |
| **Patient characteristics at the start of the study** | 15 | Table of demographic and clinical characteristics | Yes, detailed table available. |
| **Number of subjects/patients analysed** | 16 | Number of participants in the analysis | All remaining participants analysed. |
| **Results and estimation methods** | 17a | Results for each group and estimated effect size | Yes, results given with confidence intervals. |
| | 17b | Absolute and relative effect sizes | Relative effect sizes not specified. |
| **Additional analyses** | 18 | Results of subgroup and adjusted analyses | Yes, subgroup analyses performed. |
| **Damage** | 19 | All important damage (undesirable effects) | Not reported. |
| **Discussion** | | | |
| **Limitations** | 20 | Study limitations with indication of potential bias | Yes, small sample size mentioned as main limitation. |
| **Generalisability** | 21 | Generalisability (external validity) | Discussion of the results and their relevance for a broader population available. |
| **Interpretation** | 22 | Interpretation consistent | Yes, consistent |

| | | | |
|---|---|---|---|
| | | with the results | interpretation. |
| **Other information** | | | |
| **Registration** | 23 | Registration number and name of the study registry | ChiCTR1900020746. |
| **Protocol** | 24 | Where the minutes can be viewed | Not specified. |
| **Financing** | 25 | Sources of financing | Yes, comprehensive description of the financing and the institutions involved. |

### Results of the individual studies (Tables 30-62)

The following descriptions and tables (30-62) supplement section **5.5.2 Results of the individual studies**. They provide a detailed presentation of the ten selected randomised controlled trials (RCTs), including the demographic characteristics of the participants and all primary and secondary outcomes. This structured presentation promotes a clear and transparent overview of the study results.

5.5.2.1 **Atan et al.,2020**

**Demographic characteristics of the participants:** Both groups were homogeneously distributed in terms of age, gender and other demographic variables, which ensures the comparability of the groups and the internal validity of the results, see Tab. 30.

Tab 30: Demographic characteristics of the participants (own presentation 2024)

| Feature | KT (Kinesiotaping)-Group (n=15) | Control group (ST= Sham tapping) (n=15) | p-value |
|---|---|---|---|
| Gender (m/f) | 7/8 | 6/9 | 0,713 |
| Age (mean ± SD) | 44,67 ± 11,26 | 49,80 ± 11,04 | 0,218 |
| BMI (mean ± SD) | 27,46 ± 3,50 | 29,61 ±4,88 | 0,179 |
| Symptom duration (months) | 11,53 ±8,33 | 10,06 ±5,18 | 0,325 |
| Symptom frequency (days/W) | 6,73 ± 1,03 | 6,53 ± 0,99 | 0,593 |
| Tinnitus localisation | 9/6 | 4/11 | 0.965 |

### Results

Primary outcomes

Tinnitus severity (VAS): The KT group (kinesio taping) showed a significant reduction in tinnitus severity (VAS), whereas in the ST group (sham taping) no significant changes were observed. This indicates the effectiveness of KT in reducing tinnitus loudness, see Table 31.

Tab 31: Change in tinnitus severity (VAS) and disability (own presentation 2024)

| Timing | KT-Group (mean ± SD) | Control group (mean ± SD) | p-value |
|---|---|---|---|
| Initial value | 7,47 ± 1,24 | 7,13 ± 2,26 | 0,108 |
| After 4 Weeks | 5,07 ± 1,33 | 6,58 ± 1,88 | <0,001* |

□ Secondary outcomes

(A) Tinnitus Handicap Index (THI): The KT group showed significant improvements in the functional subscale of the THI, indicating a reduction in functional impairment caused by tinnitus, see Table 32.

Tab 32: Tinnitus Handicap Index (THI) (own presentation 2024)

| Subscale | Timing | KT Group (mean ± SD) | ST group (mean ± SD) | Δ within the group | p-value |
|---|---|---|---|---|---|
| Functional | Baseline | 65,73 ± 10,84 | 61,06 ± 17,72 | - | - |
| | After 4 Weeks | 52,67 ± 13,02 | 59,33 ± 17,80 | -13,06 ± 6,80 | 0,001 |

(B) neck pain and disability (VAS): The KT group showed a significant reduction in neck pain, see Tab 33.

Tab 33: Cervical pain (VAS), (own illustration 2024)

| Timing | KT Group (mean ± SD) | ST Group (mean ± SD) | Δ within the Group | p-value |
|---|---|---|---|---|
| Baseline | 6,20 ± 1,52 | 6,67 ± 1,44 | - | - |
| After 4 Weeks | 3,67 ± 1,75 | 6,13 ± 1,68 | -2,53 ± 1,20 | 0,001 |

(C) Neck Disability Index (NDI): The KT group showed a significant improvement in neck function, emphasising the effectiveness of KT in reducing disability associated with neck pain, see Table 34.

Tab 34: Neck disability index (own presentation 2024)

| Timing | KT Group (mean ± SD) | ST Group (mean ± SD) | Δ within the Group | p-value |
|---|---|---|---|---|
| **Baseline** | 19,53 ±6,62 | 23,47 ± 5,33 | - | - |
| **After 4 Weeks** | 12,80 ± 5,08 | 23,47 ± 5,46 | -6,73 ± 3,45 | 0,001 |

Statistical results and effect sizes:

Tab 35: Statistical results and effect sizes (own presentation 2024)

| Outcome | Effect size (Cohen's d) | p-value |
|---|---|---|
| **Tinnitus severity (VAS)** | 1,03 | <0,001 |
| **THI** | 0,89 | <0,001 |
| **Neck pain (VAS)** | 0,97 | <0,001 |
| **NDI** | 0,84 | <0,001 |

5.5.2.2 **Aydogan et al, 2022**

**Demographic characteristics of the participants:** The two groups were similarly distributed in terms of age and gender. The p-value > 0.05 shows no statistically significant differences between the groups, see Table 36.

Tab 36: Demographic characteristics of the participants (own presentation 2024)

| Variable | Control group Mean ± SD | TENS Group Middle! SD | p-value |
|---|---|---|---|
| Age (year) | 40,08 ± 11,76 | 38,58 ± 8,97 | 0,43 |
| Gender, n (%) | | | |
| Female | 13 (56,5 %) | 15 (65,2 %) | 0,69 |
| Male | 10 (43,4 %) | 8 (34,7 %) | 0,58 |

SD: standard deviation; Chisquare test; p > 0.05

## Results

Primary outcomes

(a) Changes in tinnitus severity (dB) and VAS: The TENS group showed significant improvements in the primary outcomes, particularly in tinnitus severity, VAS loudness and VAS annoyance (p < 0.05). No significant changes were observed in the control group, see Table 37.

Tab 37: Changes in tinnitus severity (dB) and VAS (own illustration 2024)

| Evaluation -ung | Time point | TENS group (previously) | TENS - Group (to - her) | p-value | Control group (before) | Control group (after) | p-value t | Intergroup n- Mean ± SD | p-Who t |
|---|---|---|---|---|---|---|---|---|---|
| **Tinnitu s-Schwe reg rad** | Reason -line | 54,86 ± 13,44 | - | - | 55,08 ± 14,26 | - | - | -9,04 ± 2,08 | 0,13 8 |
| | After 4 Week en | - | 42,60 ± 18,16 | 0,00 3 | - | 55,26 ± 14,16 | 0,40 0 | -7,24 ± 2,78 | |

| | | | | | | | | | |
|---|---|---|---|---|---|---|---|---|---|
| **VAS-Volume** | Reason-line | 6,34 ± 1,89 | - | - | 6,04 ± 2,09 | - | - | 2,57 ± 1,03 | 0,005 |
| | After 4 Weeken | - | 3,34 ± 2,36 | 0,001 | - | 6,00 ± 1,40 | 0,800 | 1,27 ± 1,46 | |
| **VAS harassment** | Reason-line | 6,30 ± 1,86 | - | - | 5,95 ± 1,32 | - | - | 2,70 ± 1,75 | 0,047 |
| | After 4 Weeken | - | 3,21 ± 2,25 | 0,001 | - | 5,64 ± 1,44 | 0,070 | 1,53 ± 1,96 | |

(B) Changes in THI scores: The emotional and total THI scores in particular improved significantly in the TENS group. This indicates a reduction in the emotional stress caused by tinnitus, see Table 38.

Tab 38: Changes in THI scores (own presentation 2024)

| **Valuation** | **Timing** | **TENS group (before)** | **TENS - Group (to - her)** | **p-value t** | **Contra II group (before )** | **Control I-group (after)** | **p-value t** | **Intergroup n- Mean ± SD** | **p-We rt** |
|---|---|---|---|---|---|---|---|---|---|
| **THI-Functiona 1** | Baseline | 19,56± 12,29 | - | - | 22,17± 3,24 | - | - | -7,08 ± 5,48 | 0,12 |
| | After 4 Weeks | - | 14,13 ± 10,63 | 0,050 | - | 21,07 ± 4,06 | 0,500 | -10,17 ±9,8 | |
| **THI-Emotional** | Baseline | 14,45± 6,26 | - | - | 17,50± 7,30 | - | - | -8,23 ± 7,61 | 0,4 |
| | After 4 Weeks | - | 5,27± 4,67 | 0,005 | - | 16,05 ± 5,38 | 0,200 | -4,98 ± 5,96 | |
| **THI-Catastrophe he** | Baseline | 4,06± 5,69 | - | - | 10,80± 5,12 | - | - | -2,58 ± 4,30 | 0,87 |
| | After 4 Weeks | - | 3,02± 3,81 | 0,060 | - | 10,64 ± 5,34 | 0,900 | -2,9 ± 3,18 | |
| **THI-Total score** | Baseline | 38,78± 23,50 | - | - | 50,15± 13,45 | - | - | -15,41 ± 12,40 | 0,03 |
| | After 4 Weeks | - | 22,69 ± 18,83 | 0,001 | - | 48,35 ± 23,79 | 0,600 | -12,3 ± 15,17 | |

□ Secondary outcomes(c)

Changes in SF-36 subscales: The TENS group showed improvements in several quality of life aspects, particularly in physical function and vitality. The control group showed no significant changes, see Tab 39.

Tab 39: Changes in SF-36 subscales (own presentation 2024)

| SF-36 Sub- domain | Time punk t | TENS-Group e (before r) | TENS Group (according to -her) | p-Who t | Control I - group (previously ) | Control I O group (after-here) | p-Value | Inter-group n- medium worth± | p-Value |
|---|---|---|---|---|---|---|---|---|---|

| | | | | | | | | SD | |
|---|---|---|---|---|---|---|---|---|---|
| Physical he Function | Green d-line | 84,56± 18,83 | 88,04 ± 14,59 | 0,008 | 78,69 ± 26,11 | 72,17± 21,28 | 0,834 | 6,17± 7,60 | 0,05 |
| Pain | Green d-line | 49,56± 18,44 | 55,73 ± 16,04 | 0,003 | 69,26 ± 27,20 | 72,05± 24,20 | 0,291 | 9,76± 11,85 | 0,05 |
| General ne Healthy since | Green d-line | 64,65± 18,44 | 69,30 ± 16,26 | 0,002 | 59,34 ± 16,54 | 63,62± 23,40 | 0,232 | 40,35± 134,09 | 0,199 |
| Vitality | Green d-line | 49,78± 16,05 | 53,91 ± 14,45 | 0,015 | 56,08 ± 26,20 | 55,08± 26,84 | 0,769 | 24,41 ± 8,31 | 0,855 |
| Social Function | Green d-line | 58,26± 23,22 | 61,17 ± 22,78 | 0,050 | 79,89 ± 23,58 | 77,12± 64,55 | 0,567 | 0,55± 1,50 | 0,91 |
| Emotionale role | Grunt d-line | 69,56 ± 36,12 | 79,70 ± 31,37 | 0,047 | 65,70 ± 41,62 | 76,81± 29,11 | 0,057 | | |

5.5.2.3 **Delgado de la Serna et al, 2020**

**Demographic data of the participants:** Both groups were characterised by gender, age and duration of tinnitus symptoms are similarly distributed, see Table 40.

Tab 40: Demographic data of the participants (own presentation 2024)

| Variable | Exercise + education (N = 30) | Exercise + education + manual therapy (N = 31) |
|---|---|---|
| **Gender (male/female)** | 13/17 | 12/19 |
| **Age (years)** | 44.0 ± 10.5 (42.1 to 46,9) | 42.5 ± 12.0 (39.0 to 46.0) |
| **Months with tinnitus symptoms** | 17.1 ± 5.0 (15.6 to 18.6) | 17.5 ± 6.5 (15.3 to 19.7) |

**Results**

Primary outcomes:

(A) CMD pain (NRPS): The group with manual therapy showed a significantly greater reduction in CMD pain across all time points, see Table 41.

Table 41: CMD pain (NRPS), (own illustration 2024)

| Timing | Exercise + education (mean ± SD (95 % CI)) | Exercise + education + manual therapy (mean ± SD (95 % CI)) | Difference between groups (95 % CI) |
|---|---|---|---|
| **Initial value** | 5.2 ± 1.7 (4.6 to 5.8) | 5.2 ± 2.2 (4.5 to 5.9) | - |
| **After the Intervention** | 4.1 ±1.2 (3.6 to 4.6) | 3.2 ± 1.8 (2.7 to 3.7) | -0.9 (-1.5 to -0.3)* |
| **3 months** | 4.0 ± 1.3 (3.4 to 4.6) | 2.4 ±1.8 (1.8 to 3.0) | -1.6 (-2.5 to -0.7)* |
| **6 months** | 3.6 ± 1.5 (3.0 to 4.2) | 2.2 ± 1.5 (1.6 to 3.0) | -1.4 (-2.2 to -0.6)* |

Legend: NPRS = Numerical Pain Rating Scale (0-10) *$p < 0.05$.

(B) Tinnitus severity (VAS): Manual therapy led to a greater reduction in tinnitus severity, especially after three and six months, see Table 42.

Tab 42: Tinnitus severity (VAS), (own illustration 2024)

| Timing | Exercise + education (mean value ± SD (95 % CI)) | Exercise + education + manual therapy (mean ± SD (95 % CI)) | Difference between groups (95 % CI) |
|---|---|---|---|
| Initial value | 6.7 ± 1.2 (6.2 to 7.2) | 6.8 ±1.2 (6.3 to 7.3) | - |
| After the Intervention | 5.8 ± 1.2 (5.2 to 6.4) | 4.7 ± 1.9 (4.1 to 5.3) | -12 (-2.0 to -0.4)* |
| 3 months | 5.2 ± 1.5 (4.6 to 5.8) | 3.6 ± 1.7 (3.0 to 4.2) | -1.7 (-2.6 to -0.8)* |
| 6 months | 4.7 ± 1.3 (4.2 to 5.2) | 2.8 ± 1.7 (2.2 to 3.4) | -2.0 (-3.6 to -1.0)* |

Legend: VAS = Visual Analogue Scale (0-10); *p < 0.05.

Secondary outcomes

(A) Tinnitus Handicap Inventory (THI): The reduction in the tinnitus handicap indices was significantly more pronounced in the group with manual therapy, see Table 43.

Tab 43: Tinnitus Handicap Inventory (THI), (own illustration 2024)

| Timing | Exercise + education (mean ± SD (95 % CI)) | Exercise + education + manual therapy (mean ± SD (95 % CI)) | Difference between groups (95 % CI) |
|---|---|---|---|
| Initial value | 34.2 ±11.9 (30.2 to 38,2) | 36.1 ±9.5(32.2 to 40.0) | - |
| After the Intervention | 29.5 ± 12.2 (25.7 to 33,3) | 23.0 ±8.2 (19.2 to 26.8) | -8,4 (-12,8 to -4.0)* |
| 3 months | 28.8 ± 12.3 (25.1 to 32,5) | 17.1 ±7.5 (13.4 to 20.8) | -13.6 (-18.2 to -9.0)* |
| 6 months | 28.3 ±11.8 (24.7 to 31,9) | 14.4 ± 7.3 (10.9 to 17.9) | -15.8 (-19.6 to -12.0)* |

Legend: THI = Tinnitus Handicap Inventory; *p < 0.05.

(B) Craniofacial Pain and Disability Inventory (CF-PDI): CMD-related disability was significantly reduced in the manual therapy group, see Table 44.

Tab 44: Craniofacial Pain and Disability Inventory (CF-PDI), (own illustration 2024)

| Timing | Exercise + education (mean value ± SD (95 % CI)) | Exercise + education + manual therapy (mean ± SD (95 % CI)) | Difference between groups (95 % CI) |
|---|---|---|---|
| Initial value | 38.6 ± 5.5 (36.1 to 41,1) | 40.7 ± 8.2 (37.2 to 44.2) | - |
| After the Intervention | 35.2 ± 5.0 (33.2 to 37,2) | 33.6 ±5.0 (31.6 to 35.6) | -1.6 (-3.2 to 0.0)* |
| 3 months | 34.0 ± 5.4 (31.8 to 36,2) | 29.8 ± 5.8 (27.6 to 32.0) | -4.2 (-6.4 to -2.0)* |
| 6 months | 33.3 ± 5.0 (31.3 to 35,3) | 28.7 ± 6.1 (26.5 to 30.9) | -4.6 (-6.8 to -2.4)* |

(C) Beck Depression Inventory (BDI-II): The group with manual therapy showed a greater decrease in depressive symptoms over time, see Tab 45.

Tab 45: Beck Depression Inventory (BDI-II), (own illustration 2024)

| Timing | Exercise + education (mean | Exercise + education + manual therapy (mean ± | Difference between groups (95 % CI) |
|---|---|---|---|

| | value ± SD (95 % CI)) | SD (95 % CI)) | |
|---|---|---|---|
| Initial value | 6.5 ±7.3 (4.2 to 8.8) | 7.4 ±5.4 (5.1 to 9.7) | - |
| After the Intervention | 5.7 ±6.6 (3.6 to 7.8) | 4.1 ±4.9 (2.0 to 6.2) | -2.5 (-4.0 to -1.0)* |
| 3 months | 6.3 ± 7.0 (4.2 to 8.4) | 3.1 ±4.6 (1.0 to 5.2) | -4.1 (-6.3 to -2.0)* |
| 6 months | 6.0 ± 7.0 (4.0 to 8.0) | 2.4 ± 3.8 (0.4 to 4.4) | -4.5 (-7.0 to -2.0)* |

Legend: SF-12 = Short Form-12 Health Survey; *p < 0.05

(D) Health-related quality of life (SF-12): No significant differences in health-related quality of life were found between the groups, see Tab. 46.

Tab 46: Health-related quality of life (SF-12), (own presentation 2024)

| Timing | Exercise + education (mean ± SD (95 % CI)) | Exercise + education + manual therapy (mean ± SD (95 % CI)) | Difference between groups (95 % CI) |
|---|---|---|---|
| Initial value | 31.3 ±3.4 (30.0 to 32.6) | 30.0 ±3.6 (28.7 to 31.3) | - |
| After the Intervention | 31.9 ±2.2 (30.8 to 33.0) | 30.0 ±3.4 (28.8 to 31.2) | 0.6 (-2.2 to 1.0) |
| 3 months | 32.0 ±2.5 (31.0 to 33.0) | 30.5 ± 2.7 (29.6 to 31.4) | -0.2 (-2.0 to 1.6) |
| 6 months | 31.9 ± 2.8 (30.9 to 32.9) | 30.9 ± 2.4 (29.9 to 31.9) | 0.3 (-1.5 to 2.1) |

5.5.2.4 **Eladl et al, 2022**

**Demographic data of the participants:** The groups were demographically homogeneous, with no significant differences in age, gender or affected side (P > 0.05), see Tab 47.

Tab 47: Demographic data of the participants (own data 2024)

| Parameters | Group A (mean ± SD / n, %) | Group B (mean ± SD / n, %) | P-Value |
|---|---|---|---|
| Age (years) | 41,25 ±7,22 | 40,8 ± 8,08 | 0,85 |
| Gender - Male | 13 (65%) | 10 (50%) | 0,33 |
| Gender - Female | 7 (35%) | 10 (50%) | |
| Affected parties - Bilateral | 15 (75%) | 17 (85%) | 0,42 |
| Affected pages - One-sided | 5 (25%) | 3 (15%) | |

**Results**

□ Primary outcomes

Mean VAS: Group A showed a significantly greater reduction in VAS values compared to group B (P < 0.05), see Table 48.

Tab 48: Mean VAS of the participants (own presentation 2024)

| Time of measurement | Group A (mean ± SD) | Group B (mean ± SD) | Mean difference (95% CI) | P-Value |
|---|---|---|---|---|
| Pre-treatment | 7,44 ± 0,69 | 7,25 ±0,71 | 0,19 (-0,25:0,64) | 0,38 |
| Aftercare | 3,6 ± 0,82 | 5,65 ± 1,13 | -2,05 (-2,68:-1,41) | 0,001 |
| Difference | 3,84 (3,3:4,38) | 1,6 (1,05:2,14) | | 0,001 |

□ Secondary outcomes

(A) THI values: Group A had a significantly greater improvement in THI values compared to Group B (P < 0.05), see Table 49.

Tab 49: THI values of the participants (own presentation 2024)

| Time of measurement | Group A (mean ± SD) | Group B (mean ± SD) | Medium Difference (95 per cent KI) | P-Value |
|---|---|---|---|---|
| **Pre-treatment** | 46,3 ±7,61 | 45,9 ± 8,23 | 0,4 (-4,67:5,47) | 0,87 |
| **Aftercare** | 31,05 ±4,43 | 36,4 ± 5,4 | -5,35 (-8,51: 2,19) | 0,001 |
| **Difference** | 15,25 (11,77:18,73) | 9,5 (6,01:12,98) | | 0,001 |

(B) Mean neck ROM: Group A showed a significantly greater improvement in cervical ROM parameters compared to group B (P < 0.05), see Table 50.

Table 50: Mitterer Hals-Rom (own illustration 2024)

| Parameters | Group A Before | Group A Aftermath | Group B Before | Group B Aftermath | Differentiate z A (95% CI) | Differentiate z B (95% CI) | P-Value |
|---|---|---|---|---|---|---|---|
| **Diffraction** | 40,1 ± 5,3 | 50 ±2,1 | 39,75 ± 4,17 | 46,35 ± 3,89 | -9,9 (12,03:7,76) | -6,6 (8,73:4,46) | 0,00 1 |
| **Stretching** | 53,85 ± 14 | 74,75 ± 6,38 | 54,8 ± 9,83 | 68,2 ± 9,55 | -20,9 (26,19:15,6) | - 13,4(18,69:8,1) | 0,00 1 |
| **Infringement of the law** | 36,95 ± 4,12 | 44,55 ± 1,27 | 35,8 ± 3,63 | 40,75 ± 2,53 | -7,6 (9,44:5,75) | -4,95 (6,79:3,1) | 0,00 1 |
| **Left bend** | 36,2 ± 4,55 | 43,65 ± 2,2 | 36,25 ± 3,64 | 41,9± 2,63 | -7,45 ( 9,01: 5,89) | -5,65 ( 7,21: 4,09) | 0,00 1 |
| **Clockwise rotation** | 62,1 ± 8,38 | 70 ± 1,62 | 60,6 ± 9,08 | 66,5 ± 4,61 | -7,9 (11,27:4,52) | -5,9 (9,27:2,52) | 0,00 3 |
| **Anticlockwise rotation** | 62,7 ± 7,06 | 70,25 ± 2,55 | 60,8 ± 6,23 | 67,5 ± 3,8 | -7,55 ( 10,35: 4,74) | -6,7 ( 9,5: 3,89) | 0,01 |

5.5.2.5 **Fobbe et al, 2022**

**Demographic data of the study participants:** The demographic data show a relatively balanced gender distribution with a slight female predominance. Tinnitus duration, characteristics and localisation were similarly distributed in both groups. In addition, the THI and DHI values initially show moderate impairment, see Table 51.

Tab 51: Demographic data of the study participants (own presentation 2024)

| Variable | Intervention group (IG) | Control group (KG) | Total |
|---|---|---|---|
| **Number of participants** | 37 (patients who received manual therapy ) | 33 (patients without intervention beforeT1) | 70 |
| **Average age** | 48.4 years (SD 13) | - | 48.4 years |
| **Proportion of women** | 61,4% (43) | - | 61,4 % |
| **Tinnitus duration** | < 3 months: 10%, > 10 years: 30 % | - | 3 3 months: 10 %, > 10 years: 30 % |
| **THI MW (Std. deviation)** | 43,0(19,0) | - | - |

| | | | |
|---|---|---|---|
| **DHI MW (Std. deviation)** | 32,9(16,2) | - | - |
| **Localisation** | Right: 11.4 %, Left: 27.1 %, Both sides: 61.4 % | - | Right: 11.4 %, Left: 27.1 %, Both sides: 61.4 % |

## Results

□ Primary outcomes:

(A)THI (Tinnitus Handicap Inventory): The IG showed a significant improvement in the THI from 43.0 to 22.3 (p < 0.001), while the KG changed only slightly from 45.6 to 41.6. The proportion of patients with mild THI increased in the IG from 8.1 % to 51.4 %, see Table 52.

Tab 52: THI values (own presentation 2024)

| **Timing** | **Description of the** | **IG (M ± SD)** | **KG (M ± SD)** | **p-value** | **Effect size** (r) |
|---|---|---|---|---|---|
| **T0** | Initial values before therapy | 43,0 ± 19,0 | 45,6 ± 21,72 | 0,423 | - |
| **T1** | After completion of the manual therapy | 22,3 ± 21,72 | 41,6 ± 21,72 | < 0,001 | 0,47 |

Tab 53: THI category (distribution in %) - improvement from T0 to T1 (own presentation 2024)

| **Category** | **IG T0** | **IG T1** | **KG T0** | **KG T1** |
|---|---|---|---|---|
| **Grade 1 : light** | 8,1 | 51,4 | 6,1 | 9,1 |
| **Grade 2: mild** | 35,1 | 27,0 | 36,4 | 36,4 |
| **Grade 3: moderate** | 40,5 | 16,2 | 30,3 | 33,3 |
| **Grade 4: heavy** | 16,2 | 5,4 | 18,2 | 9,1 |
| **Grade 5: catastrophic** | 0,0 | 0,0 | 9,1 | 12,1 |

(B) Dizziness Handicap Inventory (DHI): The IG showed a significant reduction in the DHI from 32.9 to 12.8 points (p = 0.01), with an increase in the mild DHI from 38.5 % to 84.6 %. In contrast, the KG showed only minimal changes, see Table 54.

Tab 54: Dizziness Handicap Inventory (DHI), (own illustration 2024)

| **Timing** | **Description of the** | **IG (M ± SD)** | **KG (M ± SD)** | **p-value** | **Effect size** (r) |
|---|---|---|---|---|---|
| **T0** | Initial values before therapy | 32,9 ± 16,2 | 31,7± 16,26 | 0,579 | - |
| **T1** | After completion of the manual therapy | 12,8 ± 20,7 | 31,1 ± 20,7 | 0,01 | 0,49 |

Tab 55: DHI category (distribution in %) - improvement from TO to T1 (own presentation 2024)

| **Category** | **IG T0** | **IG T1** | **KG T0** | **KG T1** |
|---|---|---|---|---|
| **Mild** | 38,5 | 84,6 | 46,2 | 53,8 |
| **Moderate** | 61,5 | 15,4 | 46,2 | 38,5 |
| **Heavy** | 0,0 | 0,0 | 7,7 | 7,7 |

Secondary outcomes

Tone of the neck muscles: reduction of hypertonia in relevant muscles in the IG. These results show the effectiveness of manual therapy on muscular tension, see Table 56.

Tab 56: Target parameters (muscular hypertension), (own illustration 2024)

| Muscle | Description of the | Hypertension T0 IG (%) | Hypertension T1 IG (%) | p-value | Effect size (Phi) |
|---|---|---|---|---|---|
| **M. splenius capitis (R)** | Initial and final values of hypertension | 78 | 32 | < 0,001 | 0,56 |
| **M. semispinalis capitis (R)** | Initial and final values of hypertension | 81 | 21 | < 0,001 | 0,57 |
| **M. trapezius (R)** | Initial and final values of hypertension | 85 | 40 | < 0,001 | 0,42 |

5.5.2.6 **Michiels et al, 2016**

**Demographic data of the participants:** The demographic data show no significant differences between the groups at the start of the study. The mean TFI scores were 50 and 51 points, indicating severe tinnitus impairment. The NBQ scores showed neck discomfort in both groups (37 and 32 points respectively), confirming the target population, see Tab 57.

Tab 57: Demographic data of the participants (own presentation 2024)

| Variable | Sof o rtsta rtg ru p pe (SSG) | Delayed start group (VSG) | Total | p-value |
|---|---|---|---|---|
| **Number of test subjects** | 19 | 19 | 38 | 1,00 |
| **Average age** | 46 years (±14) | 52 years (±12) | 50 years | 0,26 |
| **TFI (mean ± SD)** | 50 (±23) | 51 (±18) | 49 (±21) | 0,91 |
| **NBQ (mean ± SD)** | 37 (±10) | 32 (±12) | 32 (±12) | 0,15 |
| **VAS tinnitus** | 6 (±2) | 5 (±2) | 5 (±2) | 0,55 |
| **Hyperacusis** | 20 (±9) | 19 (±9) | 19 (±9) | 0,88 |
| **Manual rotation + AST** | 68 % | 37 % | 53 % | 0,05 |
| **AST** | 74 % | 53 % | 63 % | 0,18 |
| **Trigger points** | 79 % | 84 % | 82 % | 0,68 |
| **Provocation from Tinnitus** | 11 % | 11 % | 11 % | 1,00 |

**Results**

□ Primary outcomes:

Changes in TFI (Tinnitus Function Index) and NBQ (Neck Bournemouth questionnaire): The significant reduction in TFI in improved patients by 11.89 points after treatment (p = 0.02) and by 16.89 points after follow-up (p = 0.001) emphasises the effectiveness of cervical physiotherapy. The NBQ values showed a reduction of 18.32 points directly after treatment and a sustained improvement of 6.38 points after follow-up, see Table 58.

Table 58: Changes in TFI and NBQ (own illustration 2024)

| Timing | Change in the TFI | p-value | Change in the NBQ | p-value |
|---|---|---|---|---|
| **Follow-up treatment (T1)** | +0.67 (±4.78) not improved | 0,02 | -15.19 (±17.17) not improved | 0,57 |
| | -11.89 (±21.43) improved | | -18.32 (±15.03) improved | |

| | | | | |
|---|---|---|---|---|
| **Follow-up (T2)** | +2.42 (±8.28) not improved | 0,001 | -13.07 (±18.28) not improved | 0,41 |
| | -16.89 (±26.56) improved | | -6.38 (±24.63) improved | |

Secondary outcomes:
Global perceived effect (GPE): Immediately after treatment, 53% of patients reported a significant improvement in tinnitus impairment. This effect was still detectable in 24% of patients after 6 weeks and confirms the lasting effect of the intervention, see Table 59.

Tab 59: Global perceived impact (GPE), (own illustration 2024)

| **Timing** | **Description of the** | **SSG (n = 19)** | **VSG (n = 19)** | **Total (n = 38)** |
|---|---|---|---|---|
| **T1** | Improvement after completion of treatment | 58 % (11/19) | - | 53 % (20/38) |
| **T2** | Improvement after 6 weeks of follow-up | 24 % (9/19) | - | 24 % (9/38) |

5.5.2.7 **Plaza-Monzano et al, 2020**

**Demographic data of the participants:** The demographic data and baseline values showed no significant differences between the groups (p>0.05), see Tab 60.

Tab 60: Demographic data of the participants (own presentation 2024)

| **Feature** | **Exercise/training (n=30)** | **Exercise/training + manual therapy (n=31)** | **Total (n=61)** | **p-value** |
|---|---|---|---|---|
| **Gender (men/women)** | 14/16 | 15/16 | 29/32 | 0,850 |
| **Age (years)** | 45,8 ± 13,4 | 46,2 ± 12,8 | 46,0 ± 13,0 | 0,920 |
| **Initial tinnitus severity (VAS)** | 6,8± 1,5 | 6,7 ±1,4 | 6,7 ±1,4 | 0,880 |
| **Output THI** | 45,3 ± 12,1 | 46,0 ± 12,8 | 45,7 ± 12,4 | 0,790 |
| **PPT-Temporalis-Muscle (kg/cm$^2$)** | 1,3 ± 0,5 | 1,2 ± 0,4 | 1,3 ± 0,4 | 0,620 |

**Results**

Primary outcomes:
Tinnitus severity (VAS) and THI (Tinnitus Handicap Index): Combination therapy showed a significantly greater reduction in tinnitus severity (VAS) after 6 months (-3.1 ± 1.2 points) compared to exercise/training (-1.6 ± 0.9 points, p=0.002). The THI was similar (p<0.001), see Table 61.

Tab 61 : VAS and THI of the participants (own presentation 2024)

| **Tar measurement time** | **Movement/training (change)** | **Movement/training + manual therapy (change)** | **p- value** |
|---|---|---|---|
| **Tinnitus severity (VAS, 3 months)** | -1,2 ± 0,7 | -2,4 ± 1,0 | 0,001 |
| **Tinnitus severity (VAS, 6 months)** | -1,6 ±0,9 | -3,1 ± 1,2 | 0,002 |
| **THI (3 months)** | -5,8 ±4,1 | -12,3 ±5,6 | <0,001 |
| **THI (6 months)** | -7,9 ± 5,2 | -15,8 ± 6,3 | <0,001 |

Secondary outcomes:

PPTs over the temporalis muscle and improvements in quality of life (SF- 12): Pressure pain thresholds (PPTs) over the temporalis muscle improved significantly more in the combination therapy (+0.7 ± 0.3 kg/cm$^2$) than in the exercise/training group (+0.3 ± 0.2 kg/cm2, p=0.005). Quality of life (SF-12) increased by +8.9 ± 4.2 points in the combination therapy group, compared with +5.8 ± 3.5 points in the exercise/training group (p=0.020), see Table 62.

Tab 62: The PPTs over the temporalis muscle and SF-12 (own illustration 2024)

| Time of measurement | Movement/training (change) | Movement/training + manual therapy (change) | p-value |
|---|---|---|---|
| **PPT Temporalis (kg/cm$^2$, 3 months)** | +0,2 ±0,1 | +0,5 ±0,2 | 0,010 |
| **PPT Temporalis (kg/cm$^2$, 6 months)** | +0,3 ±0,2 | +0,7 ±0,3 | 0,005 |
| **SF-12 (6 months)** | +5,8 ±3,5 | +8,9 ±4,2 | 0,020 |
| **BDI-II (depression values, 6 months)** | -3,4 ± 2,1 | -5,6 ± 3,0 | 0,015 |

5.5.2.8 **Tutar et al, 2020**

**Demographic data of the participants:** The demographic characteristics of the participants show no significant differences between the groups (p > 0.05). This indicates that the randomisation was successful and the groups are comparable, see Tab 63.

Tab 63: Demographic data of the participants (own presentation 2024)

| Feature | Group A (n=20) | Group B (n=20) | Group C (n=20) | Total (n=60) | p-value |
|---|---|---|---|---|---|
| **Age (years)** | 41,3± 11,2 | 40,8 ± 10,5 | 41,4 ± 10,8 | 41,2 ± 10,8 | 0,920 |
| **Gender (men/women)** | 7/13 | 8/12 | 7/13 | 22/38 | 0,850 |
| **Duration of tinnitus (months)** | 30,5 ± 50,2 | 32,8 ± 48,7 | 29,7 ± 50,3 | 31,0 ± 49,0 | 0,940 |

**Results**

Primary outcomes:

THI (Tinnitus Handicap Index): After treatment, groups A and B showed significant improvements in THI compared to the control group (p = 0.001). The placebo group showed a significantly lower reduction (-9.3 ± 8.7 points) compared to group A (-27.6 ± 18.2 points) and group B (-26.5 ± 19.4 points), see Table 64.

Tab 64: THI (Tinnitus Handicap Index), (own illustration 2024)

| Time of measurement | Group A (change) | Group B (change) | Group C (change) | p-value |
|---|---|---|---|---|
| **Before the treatment** | 37,8 ±20,7 | 35,1 ±21,1 | 37,9 ±21,0 | 0,998 |
| **After the Treatment** | 10,2 ±8,9 | 8,6 ±4,9 | 28,7 ± 15,0 | 0,001 |
| **Difference** | -27,6 ± 18,2 | -26,5 ± 19,4 | -9,3 ± 8,7 | 0,001 |

□ Secondary outcomes:

Results of the secondary endpoints (DASS): The secondary endpoints (DASS: depression, anxiety and stress) showed significant improvements in all groups after treatment (p < 0.05). However, groups A and B showed significantly greater improvements than the control group, see Tab 55.

Tab 65: Results of the secondary endpoints (DASS), (own presentation 2024)

| Time of measurement | Group A (change) | Group B (change) | Group C (change) | p-value |
|---|---|---|---|---|
| **Depression** | Before the Treatment: 13.10 ± 7.89 | Before the Treatment: 13.10 ± 7.80 | Before the Treatment: 13.10 ±5.82 | 1,000 |
| | After the Treatment: 5.15 ± 5.92 | After the Treatment: 4.35 ± 2.54 | After the Treatment: 9.45 ± 5.83 | 0,004 |
| | Difference: -7.95 ± 5,77 | Difference: -8.75 ± 7,11 | Difference: -3.65 ± 3.44 | 0,013 |
| **Fear** | Before the Treatment: 13.60 ± 5.29 | Before the Treatment: 13.50 ±6.08 | Before the Treatment: 13.50 ±4.99 | 0,998 |
| | After the Treatment: 5.80 ± 3.53 | After the Treatment: 4.40 ± 3.09 | After the Treatment: 10.30 ±5.56 | 0,001 |
| | Difference: -7.80 ± 5.95 | Difference: -9.10 ± 6,11 | Difference: -3.20 ± 2,98 | 0,002 |
| **Stress** | Before the Treatment: 15.95 ± 7.10 | Before the Treatment: 15.95 ±6.04 | Before the Treatment: 15.85 ±6.23 | 0,998 |
| | After the Treatment: 8.90 ± 6.03 | After the Treatment: 6.64 ± 3.32 | After the Treatment: 12.45 ±5.62 | 0,002 |
| | Difference: -7.05 ± 5.85 | Difference: -9.50 ± 5.48 | Difference: -3.40 ± 3.58 | 0,001 |

Demographic data of the participants: Both groups were comparable in terms of age, gender and severity of tinnitus (TQ and TFI) at the start of the study. No statistically significant differences were found, see Table 66.

Tab 66: Demographic data of the participants (own presentation 2024)

| Features | Early start group (n=40) | Late start group (n=40) | Total (n=80) | p-Value |
|---|---|---|---|---|
| **Gender (m/f)** | 18/22 (45%/55%) | 24/16 (60%/40%) | 42/38 (53%/47%) | 0.168 |
| **Age (years, mean ± SD)** | 46 ± 13 | 45 ± 15 | 45 ± 14 | 0.769 |
| **Tinnitus questionnaire (TQ, points, mean ± SD)** | 37 ± 16 | 34 ± 15 | 36 ± 16 | 0.345 |
| **Tinnitus Function Index (TFI, points, mean ± SD)** | 55 ± 17 | 48 ± 15 | 52 ± 16 | 0.086 |
| **CMD pain screener (<3/>3)** | 35%/65% | 35%/65% | 40%/60% | 0.272 |

## Results

Primary outcomes:

Tinnitus Questionnaire (TQ): The early start group showed a significant reduction in the TQ score after 9 weeks compared to baseline. After 18 weeks, the results were comparable between the groups, see Tab 67.

Tab 67: Tinnitus questionnaire (TQ), (own illustration 2024)

| Time of measurement | Early start group (mean ± SD) | Late start group (mean ± SD) | Difference (p-value) |
|---|---|---|---|
| **Initial value** | 37 ± 16 | 34 ± 15 | 0.345 |
| **After 9 Weeks** | 33 ± 15 | 34 ± 15 | 0.099 |
| **After 18 weeks** | 31 ± 14 | 30 ± 14 | 0.874 |

Secondary outcomes:

(A) Tinnitus Function Index (TFI): The early start group achieved a significant and clinically relevant improvement in the TFI score after 9 weeks. After 18 weeks, the results were similar in both groups, see Tab 68.

Tab 68: Tinnitus function index (TFI), (own presentation 2024)

| Time of measurement | Early start group (mean ± SD) | Late start group (mean ± SD) | Difference (p-value) |
|---|---|---|---|
| **Initial value** | 55 ± 17 | 48 ± 15 | 0.086 |
| **After 9 weeks** | 41 ± 15 | 43 ± 14 | 0.042 |
| **After 18 weeks** | 39 ± 14 | 36 ± 13 | 0.721 |

(B) Subjective loudness (visual analogue scale, VAS): The loudness values (VAS) remained largely stable in both groups during the study period and showed no significant differences, see Tab 69.

Tab 69: Subjective loudness (VAS), (own illustration 2024)

| Time of measurement | Early start group (mean ± SD) | Late start group (mean ± SD) | Difference (p-value) |
|---|---|---|---|
| **Initial value** | 50 ±30 | 49 ±25 | 0.835 |
| **After 9 weeks** | 46 ± 28 | 48 ± 26 | 0.752 |
| **After 18 weeks** | 45 ± 27 | 46 ± 25 | 0.895 |

### 5.5.2.10 **Zhe Yu et al, 2024**

**Demographic data of the participants:** The demographic data show no significant differences between the two groups in terms of age, gender, tinnitus duration, side of tinnitus, frequency of tinnitus, PTA values, VAS, THI, NPRS and HCFA scores. This indicates good baseline comparability, see Tab 70.

Tab 70: Demographic data of the participants (own presentation 2024)

| Feature | Total (n = 43) | Immediate start group (n = 20) | Late start group (n = 23) | p-value |
|---|---|---|---|---|
| **Age (years)** | 29,02 ±6,73 (19-45) | 27,95 ±6,10 (19-43) | 29,96 ±7,23 (19-45) | 0,335 |
| **Gender** | | | | 0,820 |
| - Male | 25 (64,1 %) | 12 (60%) | 13(56,5%) | |
| - Female | 18(35,9%) | 8 (40 %) | 10(43,5%) | |
| **Tinnitus duration (months)** | 7,10 ±2,08 (4-10) | 7,05 ±2,13 (4-11) | 7,18 ±1,96 (4-10) | 0,168 |
| **Tinnitus page** | | | | 0,126 |
| - Both ears | 6(14,0%) | 4 (20 %) | 2 (8,7 %) | |
| - Left ear | 13 (30,2 %) | 4 (20 %) | 9 (39,1 %) | |
| - Right ear | 24 (55,8 %) | 12 (60%) | 12 (52,2 %) | |
| **Tinnitus frequency** | | | | 0,759 |
| - High frequency | 38 (88,4 %) | 18 (90%) | 20 (87,0 %) | |

| | | | | |
|---|---|---|---|---|
| - Low frequency | 5 (11,6 %) | 2 (10 %) | 3 (13,0 %) | |
| **PTA (dB HL)** | 20,35 ±4,52 (8-25) | 20,55 ±3,46 (13-25) | 20,17 ±5,36 (8-25) | 0,789 |
| **VAS (points)** | 3,95 ± 1,93 (1-9) | 3,65 ± 1,90 (2-9) | 4,22 ± 1,95 (1-8) | 0,342 |

| | | | | |
|---|---|---|---|---|
| **THI (points)** | 40,93 ± 16,70 (14-80) | 39,60 ± 17,94 (14-74) | 42,09 ± 16,25 (14 80) | 0,636 |
| **NPRS (points)** | 3,84 ± 2,00 (1-8) | 3,50 ± 1,91 (1-8) | 4,13 ±2,07 (1-8) | 0,308 |
| **HCFA (points)** | 19,42 ± 8,18 (10-40) | 17,75 ± 8,50 (10-40) | 20,87 ± 7,78 (10-35) | 0,216 |

**Results**

□ Primary outcomes:

Visual Analogue Scale (VAS): Tinnitus Handicap Inventory (THI); Numerical Pain Rating Scale (NPRS): The immediate start group showed significant improvements in all measured parameters after 1 week. The differences were statistically significant compared to the late start group, see Tab 71.

Tab 71: Evaluation of VAS, THI and NPRS (own presentation 2024)

| **Outcome** | **Baseline** | **Week 1** | **Δ (change)** | **p-value** |
|---|---|---|---|---|
| **VAS (points)** | 3,95 ± 1,93 | 2,40 ± 1,00 | -1,25 ± 1,59 | 0,005 |
| **THI (points)** | 40,93 ± 16,70 | 28,50 ± 14,62 | -11,10± 15,10 | 0,004 |
| **NPRS (points)** | 3,84 ± 2,00 | 2,55 ± 0,89 | -0,95 ± 1,54 | 0,025 |

Prognostic indicators: The HCFA values at baseline correlated significantly with the improvements in tinnitus scores (VAS, THI, NPRS), which emphasises the importance of somatic characteristics as prognostic indicators, see Tab 72.

Tab 72: The forecast indicators (own presentation 2024)

| **Variable** | **VAS** | **THI** | **NPRS** |
|---|---|---|---|
| **F** | 47,704 | 5,840 | 37,608 |
| **$R^2$** | 0,711 | 0,203 | 0,658 |
| **p-value** | <0,001 | 0,027 | <0,001 |
| **HCFA value** | 29,051 | 15,506 | 31,084 |
| **$R^{(2)}$ (HCFA)** | 0,596 | 0,433 | 0,613 |
| **p-value (HCFA)** | <0,001 | 0,001 | <0,001 |

PRISMA 2020 Checklist

| Section and Topic | Item # | Checklist item | Location where item is reported |
|---|---|---|---|
| **TITLE** | | | |
| Title | 1 | Identify the report as a systematic review. | Deckblatt/Titel |
| **ABSTRACT** | | | |
| Abstract | 2 | See the PRISMA 2020 for Abstracts checklist. | Seite III |
| **INTRODUCTION** | | | |
| Rationale | 3 | Describe the rationale for the review in the context of existing knowledge. | Seite 87 |
| Objectives | 4 | Provide an explicit statement of the objective(s) or question(s) the review addresses. | Seite 43 |
| **METHODS** | | | |
| Eligibility criteria | 5 | Specify the inclusion and exclusion criteria for the review and how studies were grouped for the syntheses. | 46 |
| Information sources | 6 | Specify all databases, registers, websites, organisations, reference lists and other sources searched or consulted to identify studies. Specify the date when each source was last searched or consulted. | 47,51,89-96 |
| Search strategy | 7 | Present the full search strategies for all databases, registers and websites, including any filters and limits used. | 47-52 |
| Selection process | 8 | Specify the methods used to decide whether a study met the inclusion criteria of the review, including how many reviewers screened each record and each report retrieved, whether they worked independently, and if applicable, details of automation tools used in the process. | 45-46 |
| Data collection process | 9 | Specify the methods used to collect data from reports, including how many reviewers collected data from each report, whether they worked independently, any processes for obtaining or confirming data from study investigators, and if applicable, details of automation tools used in the process. | 51-55 |
| Data items | 10a | List and define all outcomes for which data were sought. Specify whether all results that were compatible with each outcome domain in each study were sought (e.g. for all measures, time points, analyses), and if not, the methods used to decide which results to collect. | 70-76 |
| | 10b | List and define all other variables for which data were sought (e.g. participant and intervention characteristics, funding sources). Describe any assumptions made about any missing or unclear information. | 56-61 |
| Study risk of bias assessment | 11 | Specify the methods used to assess risk of bias in the included studies, including details of the tool(s) used, how many reviewers assessed each study and whether they worked independently, and if applicable, details of automation tools used in the process. | 53-54<br>62-68 |
| Effect measures | 12 | Specify for each outcome the effect measure(s) (e.g. risk ratio, mean difference) used in the synthesis or presentation of results. | 70-75 |
| Synthesis methods | 13a | Describe the processes used to decide which studies were eligible for each synthesis (e.g. tabulating the study intervention characteristics and comparing against the planned groups for each synthesis (item #5)). | 46, 56-61 |
| | 13b | Describe any methods required to prepare the data for presentation or synthesis, such as handling of missing summary statistics, or data conversions. | Kapitel 3.7.1 (s.52-53)<br>Tab 13-19 (S.70-75)<br>-Umgang mit fehlenden zusammenfassenden Statistiken oder Datenumwandlungen: N/A |

| Section and Topic | Item # | Checklist item | Location where item is reported |
|---|---|---|---|
| | 13c | Describe any methods used to tabulate or visually display results of individual studies and syntheses. | 53, 56-61<br>70-75 |
| | 13d | Describe any methods used to synthesize results and provide a rationale for the choice(s). If meta-analysis was performed, describe the model(s), method(s) to identify the presence and extent of statistical heterogeneity, and software package(s) used. | 70-75, 77-83<br>Es wurde keine Meta-Analyse durchgeführt |
| | 13e | Describe any methods used to explore possible causes of heterogeneity among study results (e.g. subgroup analysis, meta-regression). | N/A |
| | 13f | Describe any sensitivity analyses conducted to assess robustness of the synthesized results. | N/A |
| Reporting bias assessment | 14 | Describe any methods used to assess risk of bias due to missing results in a synthesis (arising from reporting biases). | N/A, da keine Studien mit fehlenden Ergebnissen selektiert wurden |
| Certainty assessment | 15 | Describe any methods used to assess certainty (or confidence) in the body of evidence for an outcome. | N/A |
| **RESULTS** | | | |
| Study selection | 16a | Describe the results of the search and selection process, from the number of records identified in the search to the number of studies included in the review, ideally using a flow diagram. | 52-53<br>Kapitel 3.2 (S.45-46)<br>47-51 |
| | 16b | Cite studies that might appear to meet the inclusion criteria, but which were excluded, and explain why they were excluded. | 52-53<br>Ausgeschlossene Studien wurden nicht zitiert |
| Study characteristics | 17 | Cite each included study and present its characteristics. | Literaturverzeichnis (S.89-96)<br>Tab 5-19 (S.56-75) |
| Risk of bias in studies | 18 | Present assessments of risk of bias for each included study. | 63-68 |
| Results of individual studies | 19 | For all outcomes, present, for each study: (a) summary statistics for each group (where appropriate) and (b) an effect estimate and its precision (e.g. confidence/credible interval), ideally using structured tables or plots. | a. 70-75 (Tab 13-19)<br>b. N/A |
| Results of syntheses | 20a | For each synthesis, briefly summarise the characteristics and risk of bias among contributing studies. | 50-61<br>Abb 3 (S. 63)<br>Tab 11 (S.64-68) |
| | 20b | Present results of all statistical syntheses conducted. If meta-analysis was done, present for each the summary estimate and its precision (e.g. confidence/credible interval) and measures of statistical heterogeneity. If comparing groups, describe the direction of the effect. | N/A bei statistischen Synthesen<br>N/A (keine Meta-Analyse) |
| | 20c | Present results of all investigations of possible causes of heterogeneity among study results. | N/A |

PRISMA 2020 Checklist

| Section and Topic | Item # | Checklist item | Location where item is reported |
|---|---|---|---|
| | 20d | Present results of all sensitivity analyses conducted to assess the robustness of the synthesized results. | N/A |
| Reporting biases | 21 | Present assessments of risk of bias due to missing results (arising from reporting biases) for each synthesis assessed. | N/A |
| Certainty of evidence | 22 | Present assessments of certainty (or confidence) in the body of evidence for each outcome assessed. | N/A |
| **DISCUSSION** | | | |
| Discussion | 23a | Provide a general interpretation of the results in the context of other evidence. | Kapitel 6: Bezug auf<br>-Côté et al 2019,S.79<br>-Buergers et al 2014, S.83<br>-Campagna et al., 2021, S.84<br>-Fabrizia et al 2024, S.85 |
| | 23b | Discuss any limitations of the evidence included in the review. | 85-86 |
| | 23c | Discuss any limitations of the review processes used. | Tab 12 (S.68-70),<br>Kapitel 6.3 (S.85-86) |
| | 23d | Discuss implications of the results for practice, policy, and future research. | Abstract, Kapitel 6.2 (S.85), 87 |
| **OTHER INFORMATION** | | | |
| Registration and protocol | 24a | Provide registration information for the review, including register name and registration number, or state that the review was not registered. | N/A |
| | 24b | Indicate where the review protocol can be accessed, or state that a protocol was not prepared. | N/A |
| | 24c | Describe and explain any amendments to information provided at registration or in the protocol. | N/A |
| Support | 25 | Describe sources of financial or non-financial support for the review, and the role of the funders or sponsors in the review. | N/A |
| Competing interests | 26 | Declare any competing interests of review authors. | N/A |
| Availability of data, code and other materials | 27 | Report which of the following are publicly available and where they can be found: template data collection forms; data extracted from included studies; data used for all analyses; analytic code; any other materials used in the review. | N/A |

*From:* Page MJ, McKenzie JE, Bossuyt PM, Boutron I, Hoffmann TC, Mulrow CD, et al. The PRISMA 2020 statement: an updated guideline for reporting systematic reviews. BMJ 2021;372:n71. doi: 10.1136/bmj.n71. 

Figure 12: PRISMA 2020 checklist (own illustration 2025)